T0243431

"For decades, Ellen Langer's work has taught us the incredible power of the mind to affect our lives. In this fascinating new book, she highlights the startling role that our mind plays in fostering or undermining what is perhaps our most important asset—our health. You will be amazed. I highly recommend this book!"

—CAROL S. DWECK, PhD, author of *Mindset*

"*The Mindful Body* presents a revolutionary and much-needed prescription for reimagining and then creating optimum health. A compelling combination of personal experience, research, and hard science, this is a must-read."

—JILL BOLTE TAYLOR, PhD, author of
Whole Brain Living and *My Stroke of Insight*

"In *The Mindful Body*, Ellen Langer answers one of the most interesting and important questions about our well-being: What matters more, mind or body? Filled with original research and thought-provoking insights, it shows that the two are not just connected but are actually one, opening us to vast potential for health and happiness."

—DAN ARIELY, *New York Times* bestselling
author of *Predictably Irrational*

"*The Mindful Body* is a remarkable work of science and scholarship, with profound implications for human flourishing. Ellen Langer's pioneering research shows that our thoughts and perceptions can rejuvenate our physical health, replenish our intellectual energy, and restore our broader sense of life's possibilities. This book offers the ultimate key to unlocking your full potential."

—DANIEL H. PINK, #1 *New York Times* bestselling
author of *The Power of Regret, Drive,* and *When*

"To call a book a 'world-flipper' sounds like the worst sort of hyperbole, but the bare facts are that *The Mindful Body* does this and more. While reading it, I loved seeing my worldview upended. But make no mistake, every semi-colon in these pages is backed up by brilliant and the hardest of hard experimental science—that has been Dr. Langer's trademark for decades. I do dearly hope we pay attention."

—TOM PETERS, author of *The Excellence Dividend*

"A fun and fascinating read from one of the world's foremost thinkers. In this practical and important book, Ellen Langer offers a host of smart tips that can lead each of us to better health and greater happiness."

—SUSAN DAVID, PhD, author of *Emotional Agility*

"*The Mindful Body* is a game changer. Drawing on provocative real-world and personal examples and fascinating original research, Ellen Langer—one of the world's leading thinkers—shows us how to unlock the full potential of our bodies through the power of our minds. This book is a must-read for anyone seeking to live a truly happy, healthy life."

—DAVID EDWARDS, professor at
Johns Hopkins Medical School

"Ellen Langer's pioneering research put mindfulness on the map in psychology and overturned our assumptions about the mind-body connection. In this engaging book, she introduces provocative ideas about how rethinking our beliefs and attitudes can actually improve our health and happiness."

—ADAM GRANT, #1 *New York Times* bestselling author of *Think Again* and host of the TED podcast *Re:Thinking*

THE
MINDFUL
BODY

THE
MINDFUL
BODY

THINKING OUR WAY
TO CHRONIC HEALTH

Ellen J. Langer

BALLANTINE BOOKS

NEW YORK

Published in the United States by Ballantine Books, an imprint of
Random House, a division of Penguin Random House LLC, New York.

BALLANTINE is a registered trademark and the colophon is
a trademark of Penguin Random House LLC.

Grateful acknowledgment is made to Zoë Lewis for permission to reprint lyrics
from "Never Too Old to Be Young," from the CD *A Cure for Hiccups* by Zoë Lewis.
Reprinted by permission.

LIBRARY OF CONGRESS CATALOGING-IN-PUBLICATION DATA
Names: Langer, Ellen J., author.
Title: The mindful body: thinking our way to chronic health /
by Ellen J. Langer.
Description: New York: Ballantine Group, 2023.
Identifiers: LCCN 2022049482 (print) | LCCN 2022049483 (ebook) |
ISBN 9780593497944 (hardcover) | ISBN 9780593497951 (ebook)
Subjects: LCSH: Mindfulness (Psychology) | Mind and body. |
Thought and thinking.
Classification: LCC BF637.M56 L36 2023 (print) | LCC BF637.M56 (ebook) |
DDC 158.1/3—dc23/eng/20230415
LC record available at https://lccn.loc.gov/2022049482
LC ebook record available at https://lccn.loc.gov/2022049483

Printed in the United States of America on acid-free paper

randomhousebooks.com

4 6 8 9 7 5 3

Book design by Jo Anne Metsch

I dedicate this book to Emmett and Theo.

Contents

Introduction

When she was fifty-six, my mother was diagnosed with breast cancer. The disease had taken over her body, and she was warned that her treatment would be complex and brutal. Her prognosis was grim from the start. Her bout with cancer—from the lump she first found under her arm to its spread to her pancreas—was difficult for her and scary for me.

According to the doctors, she had only a few more months to live. Still, I stubbornly tried to keep her spirits up and pretended that the nightmare would pass. A colleague of mine once said that I marked the edge of the optimism continuum. Perhaps that's a polite way of saying that I was in denial. (I don't believe in denial, but more about that later.)

Then the most amazing thing happened: My mother's cancer vanished.

At first, we were all elated. But I soon realized the toll the treatment had taken on her. Because she wasn't supposed to survive, the doctors hadn't worried about her life after cancer. Not having had her limbs exercised while she was in the hospital, she was too weak to walk once she returned home and was confined to a wheelchair, which made her feel even less healthy.

I was struck by how people treated her. While I saw my mother's recovery as a testament to her strength, everyone else saw only her persistent weakness. In their eyes, she was still sick, clinging to life. They assumed the cancer would come back and she'd be back in the hospital before long. They were right. Within nine months, cancer appeared, and she slipped into a coma. She was fifty-seven when she died.

Many ideas about cancer, including its treatment, have changed over the years. Now it is more often thought of as a chronic disease, not the dreaded unspeakable death sentence it was decades ago. Oncology wards may have nutritionists on staff, along with social workers to attend to emotional needs. But some things have not changed, and cancer is still predominantly treated as a disease where one's psychology is not as important as medical interventions. Yet diagnoses, while useful, direct attention to only a fraction of lived experience. Context influences our physical responses but is often overlooked by the medical world and ourselves.

I could see how this dramatically affected my mother's state of mind. I watched as the world of medicine took away her sense of control, how it made her feel sick and weak even when the cancer was gone. I saw how the diagnosis became a label that defined the way she was treated by doctors, nurses, and people outside the hospital. My mother was no longer the vivacious, beautiful woman I'd known my entire life. She was a helpless cancer patient anxiously awaiting whatever treatment the medical world would try next.

My mother's experience with cancer convinced me that our current approach to health may make us sicker. Thinking about the root causes of her illness turned out to be an inflection point for my scientific career, and it profoundly shaped the mindfulness research I conducted over the decades that followed. The word "mindfulness" has become ubiquitous since my early work in the 1970s.[1] It's hard to open a newspaper or magazine, or even listen to an interview, without the word "mindful" being used. Most of this usage presents mindfulness as a condition solely of the mind and often related to the practice of meditation. But mindfulness—as my students and I have shown—is instead the simple process of actively noticing things, no meditation required. When mindful, we notice things we didn't notice before, and we come to see that we didn't know the things we thought we knew as well as we thought we knew them. Everything becomes interesting and potentially useful in a new way.

But my use of the word "mindfulness" also, importantly, refers to a condition of the body. Indeed, I believe our psychology may be the most important determinant of our health. I'm not just speaking of harmony between mind and body. I believe the mind and body comprise a single system, and every change in the human being is essentially simultaneously a change at the level of the mind (that is, a cognitive change) as well as the body (a hormonal, neural, and/or behavioral change). When we open our minds to this idea of mind-body unity, new possibilities for controlling our health become real.

Making use of the power of a mindful body is well within our grasp.

My lab at Harvard focuses on the effects of mind-body unity on our health. It's not a wet lab, where one analyzes chemicals and the like. It's just a room (now often virtual) where my students, postdocs, and other interested faculty meet to explore unusual ideas. The members of my lab and I first tested the idea of mind-body unity more than forty years ago in what came to be known as my counterclockwise study.[2] In that experiment, elderly men lived for a week as if they were their younger selves. We housed them in a retreat that was retrofitted to suggest that time had gone backward twenty years. From the magazines on the coffee table to the albums next to the record player, from the dishes in the kitchen cabinets to the shows available (on VCR tape) on the old box TV, everything cued the sense that it was an earlier time, and that the inhabitants of the house were younger. We also asked the men to behave like younger versions of themselves. To wit, even the very oldest and those with limited mobility had to carry their own luggage up the front steps and into their rooms. If that meant they had to take one shirt instead of one piece of luggage at a time, so be it. The results of this time-machine living—of imagining themselves being their younger selves—were stunning. The men's bodies changed. Their vision, hearing, strength, and even objective appearance improved.

The findings were so at odds with the prevailing view of mind-body dualism and what was believed to be possible, that it was not surprising that some didn't believe them. Nevertheless, I was so energized by this experiment and the way in which the results so elegantly demonstrated mind-body unity that I've been exploring the concept ever since. I was emboldened to test all sorts of seemingly extreme hypotheses related to it—from how our thoughts may give us a cold, to how they control our insulin levels and the amount of sleep we need, to how they can provide a psychological cure for many chronic diseases.

The goal of all my work has always been to find out just how important psychology is to our health, and to return the control over our bodies back to us. I've set out to show that the mind is a primary determinant of the body's health, and that simple interventions to change the way we think can dramatically improve our well-being. Perhaps most important among these is my work on attention to symptom variability, where I've shown that chronic diseases such as MS and Parkinson's, as well as chronic pain, may be helped with a psychological intervention.

In the pages that follow I will unpack this thinking. But to change our minds in order to change our bodies, we first need to clear up a few misconceptions. Toward that end, chapters 1 through 5 address what I consider to be foundational issues about rules, risk, prediction, decision-making, and social comparing. If we can adopt a new view of these concepts, we are well on our way to being more mindful, confident, and empowered. My work shows that when we make these shifts in our thinking, our relationships with others and ourselves improve, and our stress lessens, all in the service of improving our health.

Chapters 6, 7, and 8 explore possibilities for our health and well-being—possibilities to which we have previously been blind. Based on mind-body research by myself and others, these chapters chart a path to a different way of living our lives—with a mindful body—and to the restoration of some of the health we've lost because of our old ways of thinking.

My work on *The Mindful Body* has taken some unexpected—sometimes bizarre—turns. Rather than ignore them, I struggle to understand them. This has led me to explore such things as mindful contagion. As we'll see in chapter 9, my early research on the topic suggests that just being in the presence of someone mindful increases our own mindfulness, which has ramifications for heavy drinkers and even those on the spectrum. I also believe that the future holds the possibility of creating a mindful utopia, and imagining that future helps us think differently about the present.

Throughout these pages, I hope to make you see that every thought we have may affect our health. Indeed, better health for all of us may be just a thought away.

THE
MINDFUL
BODY

CHAPTER 1

Whose Rules?

Any fool can make a rule. And any fool will mind it.
—HENRY DAVID THOREAU

Rules are important but, in my view, they should guide not govern our behavior. We need to take a closer look at the creation and adherence to "rules" in general before we can more fully understand the problem mindless compliance to rules has on our health.

Consider a simple, low-stakes example. I've been painting for decades, though I've never been formally trained. When I started to paint, I had no idea what the rules were. I didn't even know there *were* rules. Had I known, I think my own technique would have taken a different form. I am still amused when I go into an art supply store and see the labels indicating which brush to use for which effect, as if there were no other way to achieve it—as if there were a right way and a wrong way. On occasion, I cut the hairs of my brushes to get a novel look. I'd like to think it is this originality—the desire to create something different, a work of art that doesn't resemble anything else—that makes my paintings interesting, at least to me. The novelty might not have been possible if I had rigidly followed the rules.

This attitude has defined my artistic style. One of my first paintings featured a boy holding groceries at the top of a distant hill. In the foreground, a woman sits on a bench. When I was done with the painting, I showed it to a few friends. One person commented on my "mistake," how the perspective was all wrong, since the boy in the distance was too big. I dutifully tried to "fix" things, shrinking the boy to make him look more realistic. But then I realized that the flaw is what made the painting worth looking at.

In life as in art, although we tend to praise rule followers, I believe that breaking the rules is often necessary. Too often, we follow rules mindlessly. We buy the "right" brushes and wear the "right" clothes and ask the "appropriate" questions. When we approach the rules mindfully, however, we realize they are often arbitrary and don't make sense. You don't need to use that brush or obey the rules of perspective. It's your painting. It's your life.

That's okay with paintbrushes, you might say, but not so with health. Indeed, when it comes to our health, some people are loath to question rules created by doctors or researchers— who are we to question their authority, we ask? But it's important to remember that many health rules were created with people in mind who were different from who we are today, at earlier times before certain medical advances, and without attention to how much we differ from one another and how we ourselves keep changing. For example, years ago medicines were tested primarily on young men. This testing produced good data on how the medicine affected young men, but often proved problematic for older women since their physiology is different; medicine stays in the mature female body longer. Now, appropriately, prescribing doctors take differences in age, weight, and gender into account when they set doses.

In most hospitals, visitors are supposed to leave the hospital at seven P.M. On what data, if any, was this rule based? I told my mother's nurses that I intended to stay as long as my mother wanted me to stay. She was more important to me than their rule. They had three choices: change the rule, look the other way when I was there, or deal with the commotion I would create each time they asked me to leave. They chose to look the other way. When they created the seven P.M. rule, perhaps they thought it best for the patients, perhaps best for the staff. But now there is ample research evidence that social support is important for people's health, so perhaps the rule needs to be questioned.

Why, then, do we follow rules, even when they are arbitrary and hold us back? One reason is that much of our behavior is shaped by the labels that we impose on ourselves. In one telling study, social psychologist Russell Fazio and his colleagues asked people questions that led them either to consider ways they were introverted (for example, "When do you find social gatherings stressful?") or extroverted ("At what party you attended did you have the most fun?").[1] Then, they were given a short test known as the introversion-extroversion personality scale. Those who had been asked extroversion-eliciting questions saw themselves as more extroverted while those asked introverted-eliciting questions saw themselves as more introverted. Other research has shown that priming older adults with negative stereotypes about aging led to worse performance on a test of memory.[2] Subtly reminding women of their gender elicited more stereotypical opinions from them about the math abilities of other women.[3]

The good news is that it doesn't have to be this way. Consider research I conducted with one of my past graduate students, Christelle Ngnoumen. We were interested in whether mindfulness—essentially, the process of noticing—can reduce the limiting effects of rules and labeling.[4] To do this, we used the Implicit Association Test (IAT), which is based on work led by my colleagues Anthony Greenwald and Mahzarin Banaji. The IAT assesses whether people make subconscious associations between concepts.[5] In the test, people are asked to sort images and concepts, and the time it takes them to do so is measured. Their research showed that, for example, if someone associated "white" with "good" and "Black" with "bad," they were slower when asked to sort images suggesting the opposite, that is, that "white" was bad and "Black" was good. These varying reaction times reveal implicit bias.

In our study, people were asked to sort photos into piles, and they were directed to choose the categories for those piles themselves. But we gave some participants a chance to mindfully engage with photos of "out-group" members (people with whom they didn't share obvious characteristics) before taking the IAT. If someone sorts the images mindlessly, they are likely to default to the obvious categories of race, gender, and ethnicity, since these are the easiest labels to apply. African Americans in this pile, white people over here. Men in this pile, women in this one. In our "high-mindful" condition, however, we asked people to sort by novel psychological categories, such as how social each person seemed, or whether he or she was smiling. We also asked these participants to generate two new categories on their own.

This brief intervention made a big difference. When people used mindful labels—when they broke the usual rules of sorting—their implicit racial bias on the IAT decreased by half. In another experiment, white participants displayed increased empathy when primed to be mindful; after the intervention, they spent much more time listening to the stories of people who were not like them.

This mindfulness intervention works because it forces us to notice our surprising differences, which cut across the usual stereotypes. As a result, we begin to see people as individuals, and not as easily categorized members of a group. We ignore our self-imposed labels and the constraints they suggest. Not only can we reduce prejudice by increasing mindful noticing of out-group members, but I believe we can also reduce out-group prejudice by increasing in-group discrimination. In other words, by having people notice the differences among people like them, they come to see how different we all are one from the other, and out-group differences appear not so different after all. Just as noticing similarities among things that seem different is the essence of mindfulness, so too is noticing differences among things thought to be similar.

THE SOCIAL CONSTRUCTION OF RULES

Rules are not set in stone. In fact, laws, which are *even* firmer, are mutable and need to be questioned rather than blindly followed. Legality is not the same thing as morality. In the past, by law, women were property, and homosexuality and interracial marriages were outlawed, as was alcohol during Prohibition. In 1830, a man was beaten up because he had a beard and then jailed for defending himself. When he died forty-five years later, beards were in fashion.

Even today there are laws in some parts of the United States that are more than strange and that point out the absurdity of mindless adherence to arbitrary rules. For instance, it's illegal for a donkey to sleep in a bathtub in Arizona, illegal to have a couch on your porch in Colorado, and in Maryland it's illegal to wear sleeveless shirts in public parks. This one is my favorite: In Massachusetts it's illegal to tell fortunes without a license.

The same is true in other countries. It's illegal to sell chewing gum in Singapore, to wear heels in the Acropolis of Athens, to feed pigeons in Venice, and to run out of gas on the Autobahn in Germany. Most absurdly, Poland outlawed Winnie-the-Pooh as a mascot in playgrounds and schools because he doesn't wear pants.

One of the best ways to develop a mindful relationship to rules is to remember that rules—whether written or just culturally understood—are made by people just like us. When Adam Grant, now a professor at the Wharton School of Business, was a student of mine at Harvard, we set out to study the social construction of rules, and to better understand why that social aspect was often neglected.[6] We designed experiments that made participants more aware that rules are created by people. We predicted that if we did that, they would be more likely to act in their own best interest, even if it meant ignoring the rule.

In one of our studies, Adam and I asked people to imagine themselves as a patient, giving them varying degrees of detail about the situation. To one group, we said: "Imagine you are a patient in a hospital. You're on a bedpan. There's a busy nurse outside your room. How long does it take you to ask for help?" A second scenario went like this: "Imagine you are a patient in a hospital. You're on a bedpan. There's a busy nurse outside your room, whose name is Betty Johnson. How long does it take you to ask for help?"

The only difference between the two scenarios is that the nurse is named in the second one. When she is named, we found that people ask for help sooner. We used many different scenarios and, in each case, people were more likely to take action to get what they needed when we made people rather than role salient. When people are presented with a difficult situation and they become aware that the rules were created by people and not handed down from the heavens, they are more willing to try to change the situation so that it works better for them. They cast aside useless rules and rules of politeness or etiquette. In the case of the nurse, "don't bother the medical staff" was no longer followed when participants realized it was just one person requesting help from another. Adam was the perfect person with whom to collaborate on these studies, since he creates his own path rather than mindlessly following rules and conventions. During his interview for admission to Harvard, for example, he performed magic tricks rather than just discussing his accomplishments.

There is no context where mindless rule following is more damaging than when it concerns our health. Consider cancer. A biopsy is sent down to the lab. The cancer cells don't arrive with a label reading, "I am a cancer cell." Someone must examine the cells on the slide and decide if they are cancerous or not. There are some cells for which the pathology is clear. In ambiguous situations, however, one cytologist may see a cell as cancerous while another cytologist may see it differently. This ambiguity is almost never communicated, so a person may conclude that their diagnosis is obvious, when in fact it was highly dependent on human judgment. As a practical matter, this means that someone may be told they have cancer and someone with a virtually identical set of diagnostic criteria may be told they *don't* have cancer. The cancer diagnosis sets off a cascade of responses, some of which can have negative effects. Though not something we could ever know for sure, I've often questioned how many deaths from cancer are the result of patients giving up due to the premature cognitive commitment (mindset) "Cancer is a killer," rather than the necessary consequence of the disease. Regardless, we do know that diagnoses vary across hospitals, states, and countries. In some cases, one might fall into a more severe category than in others.

ALMOST COUNTS: THE HIDDEN COSTS OF THE BORDERLINE EFFECT

If you wait for a train in the food court basement at Grand Central Terminal in New York City, you'll notice a peculiar but consistent thing. Given the huge volume of traffic and customers, many of the restaurants pre-make several dishes, for example, salads. If you happen to order one exactly like a ready-made one, you will get it immediately. But if you watch carefully you'll see that each salad has an expiration time on it, say thirty minutes. One minute before expiry, this is a fully priced, ready-to-eat delicacy. One minute after, it's tossed in the trash. Restaurants are not even allowed to give it away for free, even to a homeless person who signs a million disclaimers. From nutritious to apparently deadly, in the span of a single rotation of a second hand on a clock.

An athlete misses earning a medal by a few milliseconds. A patient barely meets the threshold for a diagnosis. A law student fails the bar exam by one question. Are these people truly substantially different from the medalist, the healthy patient just below the threshold, or the attorney who just barely passes the bar exam?

Everything in the world exists on a continuum, whether in speed, size, virulence, or any other possible descriptor you could think of. Still, we create and mindlessly adopt sharp distinctions, and those distinctions change lives far more dramatically than marginal differences ever do. Indeed, all differences are arbitrary, but drawing hard lines between categories hides this arbitrariness and can be severely damaging. I call this resulting damage "the borderline effect." The examples are endless. Someone's IQ is 69 and someone else's is 70—but only the score of 70 is deemed to be within the range of normal. We don't have to be statisticians to know there is not a meaningful difference between 69 and 70. Yet once the person with the lower score is labeled "cognitively impaired," his or her life will unfold differently than the person with a one-point advantage.

Of course, the borderline effect has an impact on literal borders as well: Before the Second World War, the differences between the southernmost part of North Korea and the northernmost part of South Korea, or the westernmost part of East Germany and the easternmost part of West Germany, were negligible. Then hard and impermeable lines were drawn, and today there are substantial cultural differences, even when, in the case of Germany, an actual border hasn't existed for three decades.

The borderline effect has implications at every level of our lives. But what is most important for us are the ways it influences our health.

My graduate student Peter Aungle and postdoc Karyn Gunnet-Shoval and I tested its effects in the diagnosis of diabetes. In the diabetes study, we compared patients whose blood sugar levels were just below or just above the threshold that indicated prediabetes (that is, "high normals" vs. "low prediabetics").[7] Our initial hypothesis was that those who were classified as sicker would end up becoming sicker, even though a one-point difference in these medical scores is statistically meaningless given the natural variance that comes with testing.

When we talked to various endocrinologists, they all agreed that there was no relevant difference between someone who measured a 5.6 percent or 5.7 percent on the glycated hemoglobin test (A1c), which measures their level of blood sugar. Nevertheless, a line must be drawn somewhere, and standard medical protocol is to consider anyone with an A1c level below 5.7 percent "normal"—they are not at immediate risk of being diabetic. However, someone at 5.7 percent or above *is* at risk, and they are classified as "prediabetic." (A person who scores 6.5 percent or above is considered "diabetic.")

The problem with these labels is that they sound like definitive diagnoses, which obscure their uncertainty and hide the human element. As a result, people accept them mindlessly. And that's never good.

For instance, when we compared patients who scored 5.6 percent on the A1c test with patients who scored 5.7 percent—again, a difference that endocrinologists said was medically insignificant—we found a major difference in their ensuing medical trajectories. You might think that being told you're on the verge of developing diabetes would jolt people into action—to turn their medical fate around. The chart below tells another, tragic, story as those who got the prediabetic label ended up with soaring A1c results over time:

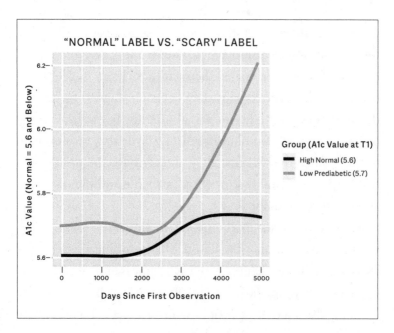

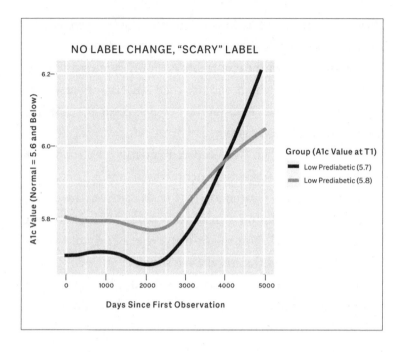

NO LABEL CHANGE, "SCARY" LABEL

Group (A1c Value at T1)
━━━ Low Prediabetic (5.7)
▬▬▬ Low Prediabetic (5.8)

A1c Value (Normal = 5.6 and Below) — vertical axis

Days Since First Observation

With diabetes at least, it would seem to be a myth that a medical scare will improve behavior. It turns out that giving people a "scary" label makes them far more likely to get diabetes down the road. Perhaps they become resigned to getting diabetes and, even after an initial attempt to eat differently, become less careful about their diets. Maybe they start exercising less, since they assume they already have the disease. Or maybe the body follows the mind, which now believes it has an early form of diabetes.

Of course, some might object to this conclusion. They might argue that the likelihood of developing diabetes increases in a linear fashion with each increase on the A1c test, no matter how small. It's a fair point. To see if this was the case, we also looked at people who measured a 5.5 percent versus those who measured a 5.6 percent. If the labels weren't driving the different outcomes, then we'd expect to see a meaningful difference in outcomes between 5.5 percent and 5.6 percent, too.

But that's not what we found. Instead, those people who were at the high end of normal tended to stay normal—the healthy label stuck. Over time, they were far less likely to get diabetes.

Unfortunately, the same was true of people at the low end of the prediabetic scale, with scores of 5.7 percent or 5.8 percent. For these patients, the exact numbers of their A1c tests were irrelevant. What mattered was the scary label, which inevitably led to scary long-term outcomes.

The difference between being labeled prediabetic or diabetic, versus just barely not, extends to insurance premiums and coverage itself. The borderline effect makes it a "preexisting condition" for one person and no problem for a virtually identical person.

There is a larger lesson here about the dangers of mindlessly consuming health information and letting the noise in data determine our fate. The language of illness, which for the most part is rooted in a biomedical model of the body (and thus ignores the power of the mind), creates an illusion of symptoms as stable and unmanageable. As a result, people quickly adopt stereotypical responses and behaviors that are in line with what they think they know, *without questioning their diagnosis and acting differently.* It is in this manner that labels corresponding to chronic conditions rob people of personal control and prevent the possibility of optimal health and well-being.

Preformed labels also encourage us to overlook our idio-syncratic experiences, which, for the most part, are never as fixed or absolute as their labels suggest. (The prediabetic should realize there is nothing inevitable about getting diabetes, provided they make small changes to their lifestyle.) But, instead, the outcome of many diagnoses of disorders can become self-fulfilling prophecies. The diagnosis creates the disease.

This doesn't mean we should never give people medical diagnoses based on their test results. Labels are inevitable. Whenever possible, however, we should ensure that our labels include a human element so patients understand that the results are provisional and uncertain.

To wit: We take an eye test or a hearing test and score right below the borderline. Hence, we are prescribed eyeglasses or a hearing aid despite our vision and hearing being virtually the same as those whose scores fell right above the borderline. And so we wear corrective devices, and they don't. What would happen, I wonder, if instead we were told the findings were probabilistic, rather than led to believe they were absolute?

Moreover, as we'll see in chapter 5, there are many temporary reasons we may perform in a certain way on a given test and then end up being put in a category requiring permanent help. It may even be that, if we took the test again the next day, our scores would suggest a very different outcome.

When we recognize that rules, labels, and cutoff points are made by people, there is lots of room to question how any situation could be otherwise. We gain a newfound sense of freedom. We expand our possibilities. This is true of our behavior, but also of our health. The key is to question those things we mindlessly accept, to mindfully interrogate all of the descriptions and diagnoses that can hold us back. When we do, we can get better. We can learn to heal ourselves.

As I discussed in the introduction, my mother's bout with breast cancer inspired most of my subsequent research. From the time she was told she had breast cancer, to her spontaneous remission, to her eventual death, she never questioned the rules she was given. I only wish I'd been able to give her this advice.

CHAPTER 2

Risk, Prediction, and the Illusion of Control

Life is either a daring adventure or nothing.
—HELEN KELLER, *Let Us Have Faith*

I go to seek a Great Perhaps.
—FRANÇOIS RABELAIS

I'm often described as a risk-taker. It's usually meant as a compliment, but to me it never feels earned. I've rarely said to myself, "This could be costly but what the hell, I'll do it anyway." Instead, I've sought approval and validation at every turn.

Case in point: When I was a junior faculty member at Harvard, I was asked to audition for a radio show. The station had a popular female psychologist host in California and wanted one for the East Coast. They called Dave Green, my department chair, for a recommendation, and he suggested me.

My audition consisted of mock call-ins. The first caller asked me a question about Rolfing, a form of bodywork therapy that involves deep massage of our connective tissue. I had about a thimble full of information on the topic but spoke with such confidence that, to my dismay, the caller asked me a second Rolfing question. Once again, I faked it well enough.

A week later I was offered the job. But after briefly thinking it over, I decided to turn it down. I didn't yet have tenure, and I very much wanted to be Professor Langer. I was worried the radio job would trivialize my work, and I was afraid I'd be seen as funny when I wanted to be seen as smart. I got tenure and continue to enjoy teaching, so I've never regretted my assessment of the risk to my gravitas I might have been taking by becoming a radio show host. Still, I have occasionally thought that had I been more mindful of what risk really is, I might have taken the job *and* soon become a professor, too. Indeed, the apparent contradiction between how I'm typically perceived by some—as a bold, risk-taking scientist—and how I perceive myself—as a somewhat risk-averse person—has led me to question some foundational assumptions about risk.

Consider an example that may clear up the paradox. When I'm at a racetrack (very rarely), I usually bet on the favorite horse to come in third—not very risk-taking. I once shared some of my confidential financial information with someone I thought I knew well, however, and as a result was defrauded out of a huge amount of money. What's going on here? At the racetrack, I take very little risk but with my personal information, I shot my wad, so to speak. While I love horses, I know nothing about horse racing, hence my conservative betting. On the other hand, I know more than a fair amount about people and thus took what might seem a big risk and trusted someone who turned out to be untrustworthy.

It's not just that we have more expertise on some things than others. Sometimes we seem to be taking a risk when we don't even realize we had a choice of how to respond. I remember being at the dentist when I was about eleven and hearing him tell my mother how brave I was. I immediately wondered what the other kids did. I didn't see myself as taking a risk in being there. I wasn't braver than they were. I just didn't know I had options.

THE MYTH OF RISK-TAKING

There is a vast literature on risk-taking. Common throughout is the belief that there are things we shouldn't do, things that are inherently too risky or not worth the potential payoff. This belief runs so deep that it rarely occurs to us to question it.

But I believe that the idea of risk-taking is misunderstood. We behave in ways that make sense to us or else we would act differently. When my expectations for success in some pursuit exceeds yours, you see me as a risk-taker. However, if you believed what I did, then you'd probably behave as I did. In other words, risk-taking is really an observer's phenomenon. "Risk-takers" do things that make sense to them, even if the same actions seem inexplicable from someone else's perspective. I'm guessing those radio producers thought I was crazy to reject their offer. Why would a junior professor turn down the chance to be famous? For me, however, the fame and fortune weren't worth the potential risk to my academic career.

Here's another example of how risk is entirely subjective. I was secretly married at sixteen. In retrospect, I can see how other people would believe that I was clearly taking a massive risk for all kinds of reasons. But risk-taking means awareness of one's own options and their potential costs. I never considered the costs. I didn't even consider other options. Gene and I—two atheists who met at a temple dance, of all things—wanted to get married, and so we got married.

It might sound pessimistic, but marriage always involves a certain amount of irrational optimism. After all, if we rationally considered the statistics—half the marriages in the United States end in divorce—we would probably avoid legally binding commitments. But when we're in love, we're not considering the numbers. We're completely convinced that our relationship is different. There is no risk of divorce, for this love will last forever.

It was initially Gene's idea to get married. He had a friend whose girlfriend was pregnant and they'd found someone in Washington, D.C., who would marry them even though they were underage. Gene was seventeen and I was sixteen at the time. We thought it would be extremely romantic to try to get the same person to marry us. On the day we decided to make a run for it, I got up at three A.M. and left a note for my parents: "Just left, see you later." Pretty clever, I thought. We drove from Yonkers all the way to Washington, D.C., in search of the person who married Gene's friend. Alas, we were unsuccessful and returned home before anyone questioned our absence.

But we were determined to get married, so Gene altered our birth certificates so that we could get married "legally" closer to home. We got the necessary blood tests. Always cautious, I made sure I was fully dressed in long sleeves, so my parents wouldn't see the Band-Aid covering the place where my blood had been drawn. Surely, as my sixteen-year-old mind believed, evidence of having had a blood test would have been enough for them to know I was newly married.

At city hall, after we were pronounced man and wife, I was given a box of household product samples. Tide, Joy, Comet, and a few other things. I couldn't stand the thought of throwing them out or refusing them, so I called home and told my mother that I just got a bunch of detergent samples. That way, she wouldn't ask me where I got them. (Didn't want to take that risk.) Later that day, I casually asked my mother for my own key to the mailbox. I would be living at home so I needed to make sure I could get the mail addressed to Mrs. Most (now my real name) before she or my father got it.

Gene and I were reasonably sure our secret was safe. Several years later, when I was nineteen, we got married again in public. I just went along with my mother's party planning and kept quiet. Before the second ceremony, however, Gene and I both agreed to admit to our mothers that we were already married. Sometime after sharing our secret, I apparently made a revealing faux pas in front of both moms, referring to the first wedding. Gene's mother knew we were already married. My mother knew we were already married. And I knew my mother and his mother knew the other knew. *So, all of us knew that all of us knew*—but when I mentioned it everyone threw me a stare making clear I was not to risk letting someone who already knew find out. I still don't know what they were trying to avoid by the deception. I do know that seeing our choice to get married as risky had the consequence of keeping us all distant from one another.

ACTOR OR OBSERVER?

Ernest Hemingway liked to tell a story about a chaotic battle fought in the Spanish Civil War. The commanding officer ordered the Lincoln Battalion volunteers to take cover to avoid enemy fire. One soldier, William Pike, didn't take cover and as a result, he was able to spot the precise location of the enemy. This turned out to be crucial in winning the battle, and Pike was rewarded with a medal for his courage. When asked why he didn't duck like the others, he replied, "I'm hard of hearing, so I didn't hear the command." In other words, he wasn't taking a risk (that he knew of), even if others were sure of it.

Blind to the situational forces that affect other people, we too readily attribute stable dispositions to them. Since the 1970s, social psychologists have studied the different ways we judge ourselves and other people. If you walk into a trash can, I may think you are clumsy. Since you know you don't always walk into trash cans, you seek a more nuanced explanation. Perhaps you were lost in thought or texting on your phone. Individuals tend to explain their behavior in flattering terms. If we screw up, it wasn't our fault—it was just the specific situation.

I go a step further, however, in my understanding of actor/observer differences. Simply put, I believe that everybody's behavior makes sense to them, or they wouldn't do it. This means that the crucial task in understanding someone else involves trying to figure out their perspective. It's not about judgment. It's about radical empathy.

Consider this scenario, which I use in my decision-making course each year: Imagine that we're in a paddock and twenty horses come racing toward us. You all run away to be safe. But I don't move. I stay there.

I ask my students to explain my behavior, and they typically assume that I must be delusional. That's when I remind them there's another alternative: While they assume the horses are going to hurt them, I think they're coming to greet me, so I happily stay put. (Say I worked on a horse farm and know that charging horses will avoid a still person.) If I thought I was in danger, I'd run, too. The point is that when people construe a situation the same way, they probably behave similarly. The important thing is to remember that there are many different ways of interpreting any given situation, even one as seemingly straightforward as twenty charging horses. I'm not in denial if I respond differently from how you would respond. I just see the situation from a different perspective. Interestingly, if I set up the situation differently and ask my students to imagine that they all stay put and I run from the horses, they instead see me as a coward.

When I was an undergraduate, I wrote something called a programmed text for my final paper in my Experimental Analysis of Behavior class. A programmed text is one that delivers instructional material in small steps with questions for self-testing along the way. It was a highly unusual final paper, and my professor applauded my "chutzpah," as he called it. Again, undeserved praise. I did not tell myself that there was risk in writing it. I thought it would be fun, so I just wrote it. If I'd known it required chutzpah, I probably would have just written a paper like everyone else.

Around the same time, my statistics professor, Gay Snodgrass, hired me as a research assistant. When I came up with an idea that she had not thought of, she was impressed and told me I was "creative." I had never before seen myself as creative. To me, that meant the kids who could draw or play a musical instrument.

Now I had permission to join their ranks. Double permission, actually—I had plenty of chutzpah and was apparently creative. Of course, had the first professor seen my response to his assignment as "ornery," or had my statistics innovations been labeled as "far-fetched," I might never have enjoyed this new sense of self and the freedom that accompanied it. Being criticized for being different would have solidified for me a sense of playing it safe.

There is a good body of research that shows that our social identity plays a huge role in our perceptions of risk. In one study, Michael Morris, Erica Carranza, and Craig Fox showed that activating people's political identities—all it took was a few questions about who they voted for—made Republicans (but not Democrats) much more likely to choose an investment option labeled "conservative" than when the options were unlabeled.[1] Although scientists have typically assumed that our risk preferences are stable, this study is a reminder that activating our "conservative" political identity can also make conservative investments more appealing.

Labels aren't just labels. They also can change how we behave. When someone gives us a label, we have several options: We can mindlessly accept it, mindlessly reject it, or mindfully consider it. If you mindlessly respond, there's no growth. You simply continue as always, stuck in the same stale categories. Mindfully evaluating the label, however, means that we don't simply consider the truth of the label. Rather, we consider the utility of the label, and what it can teach us about ourselves. When Gay Snodgrass called me creative, I could have easily rejected the label, since it didn't fit with my own self-conception. But I decided to explore the label and cultivate my own creativity going forward. And that has become a defining feature of my career.

RISK AND PREDICTION

All this points to my contention that it's virtually impossible to classify people as risk-seeking or risk averse. People continue to throw these terms around all the time, but when you stop and mindfully consider their behavior, you can't really apply those categorical labels. Again, someone who appears to you to be taking a risk—not wearing a helmet when riding a bicycle, for example—is acting in a way that seems, at least to him, to be reasonable. If you don't wear a helmet, it's not because you want to incur injuries. You just really like the feeling of the wind in your hair and, more important, you implicitly assume you won't have an accident (or get arrested in a state with a helmet law).

But the idea of risk-taking is misunderstood in another way: Risk can rarely be assessed in advance of taking action. It is not that some things are predictable, and others are unpredictable. It's that virtually everything is unpredictable, including our human reactions to events. Let's take a particularly simple scenario: I was at an event in Boston many years ago and saw a man being physical with a young girl, grabbing her arm rather forcefully and leading her toward a car. At that time I just presumed the man was the girl's father. But now, given how sensitized we've become about sexual abuse, I wonder if he might have been a predator and she might have been in trouble. Which was it? I don't know. In this sense, prediction is no different than a guess or a hunch and, as we will see, a decision is also just a prediction or guess. I had no idea what was actually happening at that point but assumed all was fine. Today I might behave differently and at least consider intervening.

Perhaps we think we can predict because we overlook the many mistaken predictions we make daily. Every embarrassment we suffer is an instance of our mistaken predictions. How often do we push or pull when we should pull or push to open a store door; reach into the silverware drawer for a knife and pull out a fork; unsuccessfully look for the sock in the dryer? In each of these scenarios we predict that our action will be successful, and we come up short. How many people predicted they'd never get COVID-19? How many of us predict we'll never really lose our strength or our ability to remember? How many of us predict we'll be fine with very little sleep? We predict these things incorrectly almost all the time. What about our inability to predict the behavior of others? How often have we waited for a phone call that never came, or came a day later than predicted?

More important, perhaps, are the predictions medical professionals make. My mother's medical team predicted she would die soon because her cancer had metastasized to her pancreas. As a result of their prediction, they didn't exercise her limbs. As noted in the introduction, this meant she left the hospital in a wheelchair, which to her suggested weakness and thus might have contributed to her ultimate death. With the cancer gone, she otherwise might have felt elated and strong. Whether we have medical training or not, we cannot predict the future. If the medical world accepted this, no matter what our conditions are or how old we may be, we would be treated with the expectation that we will heal.

Another reason we tend to be oblivious to the illusion of predictability is because of our mindlessness. This one is a bit more complicated. Imagine that someone comes over to you and is flirting, for example. You might predict that you're about to be asked out for a date. Now what if instead of thinking the person was flirting, you thought the person was actually mocking you? If asked if you thought the person would call for a date you'd surely predict no. Instead of either of these scenarios, imagine if at the start you weren't initially sure if the person was flirting or mocking you. In this case you'd be unlikely to make a prediction at all.

Every situation and every behavior can be understood in multiple ways. The more we appreciate this uncertainty, the less likely we are to make predictions in the first place. Thus, the more mindful we are of the many possibilities that exist, the more we can accept the illusion of predictability. When we see things in a single-minded way, on the other hand, it's easy to discount our misprediction. And so the illusion of predictability continues. We might say to ourselves that the flirt intended to call but got distracted by other things. In other words, the phone hasn't rung yet, but that doesn't mean it won't eventually. And thus, our presumed power of prediction remains intact.

Although most people don't readily acknowledge that predictability is illusory, there are hints of this in the culture. The most literary of these is probably Oscar Wilde who said, "When the gods want to punish us they answer our prayers." More common is the oft-stated warning "Be careful what you wish for." If the wish is fulfilled it often comes with a completely unexpected downside. In a similar vein, we speak of "unintended consequences."

Some may say that predicting has merit because at least sometimes our predictions come true. The problem here is that we can't know in advance which predictions have merit, and as social psychologist Dan Gilbert has found in many studies, even of the ones with "merit," we don't know if the outcomes will actually be as good or as bad as we anticipated.[2]

When I awoke to a rainy day when I was in junior high, I didn't want to go to school because my hair got all curly and frizzy when it rained. If you'd told me then that I'd love rainy days when I got older for the very same reason, I wouldn't have believed you. Curls are now in fashion, so let it pour. Mistaken predictions are certainly not just for children.

A wonderful surprise that I wouldn't have predicted concerned the possibility of a movie about my work. Several years ago, movie producer Grant Scharbo contacted me about doing a movie about my counterclockwise research study, the one in which we turned back the clock and witnessed that the participants looked and felt younger. Grant's wife, Gina Matthews, would join Grant in producing our movie. She had been one of the producers of *What Women Want*, starring Helen Hunt, and we all agreed that Helen would be a good choice to play me.

A few weeks later, I was shopping in the meatpacking district in New York. Who walks in but Helen Hunt. Neither of us lived in New York, but there we both were. We literally bumped into each other in the dressing rooms, so I shyly introduced myself and told her about the movie. She was more charming and beautiful than I had ever seen her on the screen.

As it turned out, Helen Hunt wasn't available to play me after all, and several years went by. Grant and Gina suggested many great actresses for the role but for an assortment of reasons, none of them worked out. Then they approached Jennifer Aniston, and things looked promising again. They arranged for me to meet Jennifer and her producing partner, Kristin Hahn, over lunch at Jennifer's house in Malibu.

When I first walked in we were all nervous. I was, after all, the big professor; she was the big star. I was taken aback by Jennifer. She literally glowed. When we got around to talking about dogs, she found a magazine with a picture of her dog in it with her. She was in a provocative pose and was embarrassed by it. Her embarrassment was my comfort. She was overwhelmingly real. I loved it. If asked in advance, I wouldn't have predicted that being genuine was a likely characteristic of an actress. My authenticity was to me the most precious aspect of me, and she was equally authentic—or such a good actress that I couldn't tell the difference. It didn't matter. They all sat on the floor around me, and I professed. It was as good as my best seminar.

We had a great lunch with easy conversation and flowing wine. When the meal was over, however, Jennifer looked a bit stressed. She awkwardly announced that she was going outside to have a cigarette. I stood up and said I would join her. Her face lit up. I said, "It's a dirty business, but someone has to do it." She said, "Yeah and I hate quitters." We left the table for the terrace and bonded.

I hoped the movie would be made. So far, many years later, it has not. For me, it doesn't matter. I live in the world of possibility, and there is always something exciting around the corner.

THE ARBITRARINESS OF INTERPRETING RISK

This raises another important issue regarding predictability that we'll see again in more detail in later pages. Whether something is good or bad is in our heads, not in events. Everything can be seen in either way depending on how we talk to ourselves. It is true that a half-empty glass is always half full. My mother died when she was young and, as a result, I have memories of her only as a vital, beautiful woman, and she never suffered the indignities that so many elders experience on a daily basis.

I'm not unusual in having had a lifetime of unpredictable experiences. What may be more unusual is that my reflections on them, after the fact, have led me to recognize the illusion of predictability.

Shortly before Christmas some years ago, a fire in my house destroyed around 80 percent of my possessions, including my lecture notes and all the gifts I'd bought for the holidays. It was objectively terrible.

The night of the fire, I arrived home from a dinner party at eleven-thirty to find my neighbors waiting outside for me.

They had waited in the cold, so I wouldn't have to face the damage alone. They also wanted to make sure I knew my dogs were okay, which was very meaningful to me.

The next day I called the insurance company. The damage was complete, I explained, but I had told myself the house held only objects, objects that reflected who I had been and not necessarily who I now was. When the agent arrived at the rubble the next day, he said, "This is the first time in my career that the call was not as bad as the damage." To my mind, the damage was already done, and it seemed pointless to add my sanity to the list of losses.

I was not quite as sanguine about losing my books and course material. At first, I thought of telling the chair of the department about the fire and asking to be relieved of teaching because I didn't have any notes to teach from and the semester would begin in just a few weeks. This surely would have been okay. Still, it would have put a burden on my colleagues, so I decided I would do what I had to do to keep my teaching commitments.

I threw myself into preparing for the class ahead. With my course notes destroyed in the fire, I contacted one of the best students from the year before and, in a twist of the professor-student dynamic, borrowed her notes to help me prepare. I also described my fire experience the first day to forewarn the students. On many levels, I was predicting the class wouldn't go well. But to my surprise, it was probably the best course I ever taught. I was totally present and focused, and the classes felt completely fresh, for both myself and the students.

In the days and weeks after the fire, my dogs and I stayed in a hotel in Cambridge. On Christmas Eve, I left the hotel to go to dinner. When I returned, to my surprise the room was filled with gifts. They were from the chambermaids, the men who parked my car, the waitresses, the clerks at the desk. Their compassion and kindness brought tears to my eyes. Although I wouldn't have predicted it then, I don't miss any of the destroyed objects lost in the fire. But every Christmas I still feel warmth when I recall the generosity of these loving strangers.

I can't be that different from everyone else, and the number of notable examples of unpredictability in my life are too many to describe. Consider one regarding my mother.

She was a banquet manager, as it was called then, arranging weddings, bar mitzvahs, and the like. Although she spent a great deal of money on clothes for the events to look different from the invited guests, on one occasion, she and the bride's mother showed up in the same dress. Who would have predicted this, given the number of dresses available from which to choose? After that embarrassing experience, she decided to have a tuxedo skirt suit created just for her. It was the first of its kind, and thus she would feel safe from a repeat performance. Again, every embarrassing moment we experience is by definition unpredicted.

My favorite example of the inherent uncertainty of events involved our dog Sparky. Sparky had clear likes and dislikes. You could never be sure how he would feel about anyone. Would he wag his tail and ask for attention? Or attempt an attack?

One day he was with Nancy, my spouse, at her store. Someone entered the store; Sparky decided he disliked her and nipped her hand. It wasn't serious, but Nancy waited for the dreaded call from the woman's attorney. She was sure she would be sued. Not so. Instead, the woman called and thanked Nancy, because Sparky had saved her life. She had been gardening and wore a thick rubber glove due to the dog bite. She hit a live wire with her gloved hand that otherwise might have electrocuted her.

We think we can predict, but all we have is hindsight. After an event, many of us become Monday morning quarterbacks. Working backward we see how it all makes sense; the dots are easy to connect. Will Jane and Bill get divorced? Who knows? Once Jane and Bill announce they are getting a divorce, we remember all the unkindness they showed each other and feel we should have known. But we couldn't have known. There were many kindnesses as well.

Predicting risk is usually impossible. When I was an undergraduate at NYU, I went to Puerto Rico with a faculty friend during winter break. While we were on the beach, my friend met two men who were sailing to the Virgin Islands. They asked us (really her) to join them on the trip. We went. I didn't realize how seasick I would become. While she was drinking and flirting, I was heaving off the side of the boat with the wind returning all I was intending for the sea. (Not a risk I foresaw.) When we landed, she decided to stay on the boat with one of the men and said she would meet me the next morning. The other man agreed to drop me off at the hotel we had chosen, but then asked if it was okay with me if he dropped me at a bus stop instead. I agreed that I would make my way from there. Unfortunately, the bus stop was directly outside a crowded bar and, although I still was coated in sand, saltwater, suntan lotion, and vomit, I was starting to get aggressive catcalls from the men in the bar.

Just then, a Jeep drove up with a young couple in it. They saw me alone, on the side of the road, and asked where I needed to go. I was now faced with a choice. Should I take the ride with this wholesome-looking pair of strangers or wait in the dark with these unwholesome-looking men staring at me? Which was the riskier choice?

I got in the Jeep with "Sundance" and "Sandy," who agreed to take me to my hotel. As we drove for some time through a jungle and away from anything inhabited, it became clear to me that the hotel was no longer our destination. I asked Sundance if we were heading to the hotel, as promised. He said he didn't know where it was but would find out in the morning.

We finally arrived at a clearing in the remote jungle. I was escorted to a giant treehouse full of people—mostly large men but a few women. These people were less wholesome looking than Sundance and Sandy. We sat in a circle on the floor, and they passed around a joint. I took a puff every third time to fit in but not get high. Someone asked me if I knew who they were and when I said I didn't, he told me they were members of Hells Angels. Trying not to reveal the fear in my voice, I asked if they would take me to the hotel in the morning. Someone asked where the hotel was and, alarmingly, Sundance answered. Clearly, he'd known where it was when he picked me up. My plan became this: Make sure they like me, so they don't hurt me. Make sure they don't like me too much, so they'll let me go.

I had no way of knowing if they really were Hells Angels or just trying to mimic them, but in either case it was frightening. I made it through the night without incident. In fact, in the morning light, the place looked like a healthy sixties commune. I got in the Jeep again with Sundance and Sandy and, as they'd promised, they dropped me at the hotel. They even drove around a few times to make sure I was okay.

Why was this experience so meaningful and memorable for me? Sure, it was terrifying. But I think it was also an introduction to the difficulty of decision-making. Should I have known better than to take a ride with strangers? They looked clean-cut while the men in the bar seemed drunk and unruly. Should I have investigated how soon the bus would arrive, if it arrived at all? Should I have known that all would turn out okay and not spent the night so scared?

Actions look risky when others deem the likelihood of success is low. My parents would have been horrified that I got into that Jeep. And yet, I also remembered the original context of the decision, which is that I was waiting for a bus outside a loud bar filled with catcalling men. When I think about those circumstances, I don't take myself to task for getting into the Jeep. At the time, it seemed like the safer option. My parents probably would have agreed if they knew the alternative I had. If we know why we did what we did, we won't have regrets for not doing otherwise. Indeed, regrets never make sense because they presuppose the alternative would have been better. Everything changes once we make a decision and take action, which means we can never know what the "road not taken" would have been like. When we are displeased with our choice, we mindlessly assume the unchosen alternative would have been better, and then we suffer whenever we think about what we may have missed. The unchosen alternative could have been better, worse, or the same. As we'll see in chapter 3, a mindful decision-making process can help us avoid this stressful cycle of regret.

But back to the Virgin Islands adventure. My choice to get into the Jeep raises another question: *Why did getting into the Jeep seem safer?* It gave me a sense of control. I had no idea when the bus might arrive. But I could control whether or not I got in the car. When it comes to risk assessments, that sense of control can make a big difference, a phenomenon that would mark the first major finding of my scientific career.

THE ILLUSION OF CONTROL

When I was a graduate student at Yale, I played in a poker game with other students, many of whom are now prominent psychologists. As with virtually all poker games, cards are dealt clockwise to each of the players. One night, the dealer skipped a person as she dealt the cards. Upon realizing the error, she gave the next card to the person who had been overlooked. People immediately objected, yelling "Misdeal! Misdeal!" Remember that the cards are dealt facedown. It was as if one of the players owned the card that no one had seen and, because it was in the hands of another player, all now would be thrown off. The way the dealer tried to correct her error seemed sensible to me, but not to most of my colleagues, despite the fact that by and large, they were a rational group of scientists.

I saw the same thing in Las Vegas where people guarded their "hot" slot machines and even engaged in intimate discussions with them. They seemed to believe they could control chance by pulling the lever one way or another, and talking sweetly to the machine.

This got me thinking about their "illusion of control," and I decided to conduct a series of experiments to document it.[3] In one, I chose to study how people play the lottery. We created two types of tickets—some that featured familiar letters from the alphabet and others that were covered in unfamiliar symbols. We then allowed some participants their choice of ticket even though while choice matters in situations where we can exercise control, it shouldn't matter in a lottery drawing. (This was before state lotteries gave people the choice of lottery tickets.) The randomness of lotteries should lead people to conclude that having a choice of which kind of ticket is meaningless.

Once people had their tickets, I gave them the opportunity to exchange them for one in another lottery with better odds. The results were clear. If a ticket had been chosen and had a familiar letter from the alphabet on it, more than four times as many people wanted to keep it. Keep in mind, this dramatic shift in preference occurred even though the odds were *better* if they exchanged their ticket.

The illusion of control can also convince people that familiarity is meaningful even in situations like games of chance, where we know it doesn't matter. Of course, experience and practice can improve outcomes in games where skill matters; on a chance task, practice doesn't have any effect. Being a slot machine addict doesn't improve your chances of a payout. Nevertheless, in my studies, I found that people who were more practiced with a game of luck were also more confident of their success in playing it.

I then wondered if people's confidence could be triggered

without their having actively participated in the chance event beyond just buying a ticket. To study this, I took advantage of a lottery conducted at Yonkers Raceway in which the entrance fee automatically enrolled you in a lottery. We approached people twenty minutes before the first, fifth, or ninth race and gave them a questionnaire that assessed their confidence in winning. The longer they had their ticket, and the more opportunity they had to think about the lottery, the more confident they were that they would win.

I tested this again in an office lottery in which some people got a lottery ticket with a complete set of numbers on one day. Others received their numbers over three successive days, so they had to think about the lottery at least three times. Once again, people were asked if they wanted to trade their ticket for one in a lottery with better odds. Those who had to think about the ticket at least three times were twice as likely to *refuse* the trade, even though, once again, trading would make them more likely to win.

Another study in this series looked at the effects of the illusion of control on competition. In a skilled competition—say, a wrestling match—your competitor would indeed matter. It would be easier to wrestle someone who weighed less, or was less skilled, just as the likelihood of winning a game of chess would depend on if you were playing against a chess grandmaster or a novice. In this study, however, people wagered on the outcome of a game that involved drawing a high card, which as a game of *chance,* was one where competence was not an issue. Some players were paired with an attractive, dapper, and confident competitor; others were paired against an awkward and nervous competitor dressed in an oversized jacket. As expected, people wagered much more against the opponent perceived to be an incompetent schnook, even though skill would have no impact on any given match.

These studies on the illusion of control were the subject of my graduate dissertation. At the time, psychologists believed that normal, healthy people were rational agents. When making choices, they assumed that people carefully compared the alternatives and maximized their utility. My research showed that people often behaved in irrational ways, rejecting better bets because of their illusion of control.

Before I could receive a PhD, I, like everyone else, had to defend my dissertation before a faculty committee in an oral exam. The oral exam for my PhD began in the typical way: I gave a brief talk about my work, followed by questions from the committee. So far, so good. Then one of the professors on the committee expressed some misgivings. I responded to his remarks as best I could and then asked him if he was suggesting there was a hole in my work. To the shock of everyone in the room, he said there wasn't a hole. "In fact," he said, "there is no doughnut." He didn't see how all the studies were tied together. The rest of the committee argued with him. Not surprisingly, I was shaken but got my PhD and remained confident in my work.

At the time, there was no way of predicting the future influence of these studies. I had no idea that they would be cited thousands of times and help dismantle the model of human rationality.

It's yet one more piece of evidence that we shouldn't put too much stock in prediction.

WHAT CAN WE CONTROL?

In the forty-five years since I conducted the first illusion-of-control studies, we have learned far more about the phenomenon. Researchers have studied who is more or less likely to exhibit the illusion and when. For example, psychologist Nathanael Fast and colleagues found that having power increases the illusion of control.[4] Thus, the wealthy and educated act as if they can control the uncontrollable. Other research has shown that this illusion can have costly consequences, as when financial traders make worse decisions when they believe they have control over the market.[5]

But I've also come to revise my own thoughts on the illusion of control. In short, I believe that the illusion of control is not always an illusion. While it might lead people to choose seemingly worse gambles in the lab, it can also help us cope with risk and uncertainty in real life. In this sense, the so-called illusion is often a necessary psychological strategy. Control is motivating, helping us handle all sorts of unpleasant and difficult situations. After all, if you believe you have no control, then you may become helpless.

In an experiment that psychologists David Glass and Jerome Singer conducted in 1972, participants were exposed to uncomfortable noise.[6] One group had a button to press if they wanted to stop the noise, but they were discouraged from using it. The comparison group was not given any means to control the noise. Neither group took action to alleviate the discomfort, but those who believed that they had control over the noise so that relief was available if they needed it had fewer adverse reactions.

Here's another example. You're waiting in an elevator. You've pressed the button for your floor, but the doors are still stuck open. Seconds pass; you can feel your anxiety building. To deal with the situation, you repeatedly press the close-door button. Then you press it again. The doors finally close.

If you're like most people, you're convinced that your button pressing made a difference. But chances are that it didn't. In 1990, the Americans with Disabilities Act mandated that all elevators must stay open for at least three seconds, so that someone with a disability has enough time to enter. In response, many elevator manufacturers deactivated the close-door buttons entirely.

Here's my point: Even if the buttons don't work, they still give riders a sense of control. They help us deal with those seconds when the doors refuse to budge. That feeling of efficacy makes a difference. Furthermore, giving people a sense of control gives them real control over the discomfort of being in an elevator that doesn't seem to be working. Even broken buttons can make us feel better.

The more important point is that, from an individual's perspective, the illusion of control is not a mistaken belief. By believing in our control, we gain real power; the "illusion" often represents an effective response to the demands of the situation. To repeat one of the important themes of my research: People act in ways that make sense from their point of view; otherwise they would act differently.

Imagine there is no illusion of control, and that people are actually quite realistic about their ability to influence random outcomes. In this alternate universe, people wouldn't care if they got to pick the lottery tickets, and they certainly wouldn't repeatedly press broken close-door elevator buttons. Sounds rational, right?

This reasonable alternate universe, however, would also create some issues. If we gave up the "illusion" of control, I think we'd also surrender real control over the mind. For instance, if we didn't press that broken elevator button, we'd have a tougher time handling those feelings of stress and impatience; our emotional control would suffer.

Or consider my vacation in Puerto Rico. When I got in that Jeep, I felt like I was taking control of the situation. Perhaps it was an illusion—I was hopping into a car with strangers, after all—but I believe that my feeling of control gave me the presence of mind to effectively deal with events that followed.

But there's a larger issue with seeing the illusion of control as just another illusion. Because there are so many unknowns about the real causes of control, *not* believing in the possibility of control would lead to instances in which we underestimate our ability to influence events. In the United Kingdom, for example, the close-door buttons in elevators work. But you'd never learn that if you assumed they were unrelated to the door speed, as many people in America think. That's why it's better to believe we may be able to control events, even if it occasionally leads us to pick suboptimal gambles in a science experiment.

Again, the illusion of control is not an illusion for the person who holds it, just as taking a risk is not a risk for the person who takes it. When people in general learn about illusions they assume they should not engage in the behavior. As we will soon see, we can experience the benefits of improved health and decreased stress by mindfully perceiving control. If we're diagnosed with a dread disease and assume we have no control, we become helpless, which itself is bad for our health.

MINDFUL OPTIMISM

One of the advantages of this approach is that it helps us focus on what we can actually control. Given the inherent uncertainty of the universe, and the limited powers of the human mind, it seems crazy to think we can anticipate every outcome and risk in advance. When we seek control *before* we make the decision, we're setting ourselves up for stress and disappointment. The much better approach is to focus instead on controlling events *after* the decision. As we will see in chapter 4, trying to predict the future is the real illusion of control. The problem with decision-making is that we tend to get stressed not only by consequential decisions but also about inconsequential choices. The impact of that stress can be worse than the worst-case scenario triggered by the "wrong" choice.

For one thing, being worried about our decision outcomes can lead to defensive pessimism, in which we continually prepare for the worst. To me this is a losing strategy. Events are neither good nor bad. It is our thoughts that make them so.

Defensive pessimism keeps us on the lookout for the negative. Seek and ye shall find. Being inundated with negative thoughts keeps us stressed, which is not good for our health. Expecting defeat too often creates defeat.

I propose we adopt an attitude of mindful optimism. This doesn't mean we should bury our heads in the sand with a certainty that all will be fine. Rather, it involves recognizing that uncertainty is not new. Neither is risk. Everything has always been uncertain, we were just oblivious to it.

We can worry or relax, and things can turn out good or bad. If we worry and everything turns out fine, we've stressed ourselves unnecessarily. If we worry and things turn out to be bad, we're usually no more prepared for it than if we didn't worry. If we relax and things turn out bad, we'll be stronger to deal with it, and if it all turns out to be fine, we can continue behaving adaptively.

How can we adopt a life strategy of mindful optimism? I was thinking about this during the beginning of the COVID-19 pandemic, as so many people were struggling with chronic anxiety and chronic pessimism. For me, mindful optimism began with implementing a useful plan, such as washing my hands and wearing a medical grade mask. It also meant that I followed social-distancing instructions. After following my plan, however, I then made a concerted effort to live fully moment by moment with the implicit expectation that all will be fine.

Indeed, if we accept the intrinsic uncertainty of life, we can adopt a more mindful perspective around rules and rule breaking. When I was in the hospital with a smashed ankle, I passed the time by painting with watercolors. One of the nurses was especially curious, so I attempted to teach her how to paint from my perspective. Rather than worry about doing it the "right way," or following the "rules of painting," I told her to just do it. I explained that for me the process comes alive as soon as I make a "mistake." I emphasized that they weren't mistakes at all but just portals into something new.

Because many people believe that art is subjective, they can readily accept this radical advice. The nurse seemed to embrace it—she seemed to enjoy having the freedom to just paint. Scientists, however, are less willing to let go of certainties. While science has an air of objectivity, we must remember that all of the variables being studied—the kinds and amount—were selected by people who have their own biases. Changing them could change the findings, which again are only probabilities, not absolutes. We should give up the idea of objective probabilities, or predictable risks, or decisions that can be classified as right or wrong in advance. Instead, we should treat all of our choices as opportunities for growth and education.

Once we do that, we'll come to see that emotions like stress and regret become less of a problem. And the world becomes a less scary and far more interesting place.

CHAPTER 3

A World of Plenty

Not what we have but what we enjoy
constitutes our abundance.
—Jean Antoine Petit-Senn

Are you a glass half-empty or a glass half-full kind of person? We hear this dichotomy thrown around in all kinds of contexts, but what this trite question is really getting at is the issue of plenty or scarcity.

A friend of mine had a gift for seeing everything in a negative light. Or at least that's how I first understood it. When I returned from shopping one day and excitedly reported that I'd found sneakers on sale, she looked glum.

I soon realized that while I thought I was sharing good news so she could take advantage of the sale, she saw the availability of shoes as a zero-sum game. In her view, if I got something, there was now less available for her. Since she lived in a world of scarcity, she assumed I had bought the last available pair of those shoes.

Some people—like me—see a world of plenty. If I hear

that someone got a good deal, I assume that I can get one, too. The underlying assumption is that there's enough to go around, and that the shoe store surely has more sneakers on sale.

Perspectives like this shape our lives. But we make matters worse by assuming that a person's sense of plenty or scarcity is stable and fixed. That is, we wrongly take for granted that if you see a world of scarcity and limits, you are bound to always see a world of scarcity and limits. Metaphorically, you will always be jealous of people who find shoes on sale. The good news is that, as we'll soon learn, our perspectives needn't be fixed at all. We can adopt new perspectives and—especially when it comes to our health and our experience of aging— when we do, our lives may improve dramatically.

IS "NORMAL DISTRIBUTION" NORMAL?

The presumption of limited resources is widely held. We believe that talent and skills, as well as material assets, are all "normally distributed." That means that some people have a great deal, most an average amount, and some very little. If we give people an IQ test, for example, and plot their scores on a graph, we'd probably see what looks like a bell. This is called the normal distribution of scores. A few people have high IQ scores, most people have average IQs and score close to the middle, the mean, and a few have low scores. It doesn't matter if you're talking about intelligence or beauty, self-control, or kindness: We assume these qualities have been allocated unequally to the population. A small proportion of people have

a lot, most of us have an average amount, and a small proportion of us have very little.

Is good health distributed normally? It seems to me silly to
think of health as being a static condition that is randomly
distributed. Yet that is the way too many of us treat our health.
Obviously, our health can improve or deteriorate. It's not random, and it's not normal. We lose a great deal when we accept
that some small proportion of people will be really healthy,
and some are destined to be ill. In fact, good health may be
equally available to virtually all of us.

Yet the concept of scarcity remains ubiquitous. The underlying belief is that we can't all have talent, smarts, beauty, and
so forth. There's a reason we call it the *normal* distribution—as
if it could be no other way. If things need not be seen as scarce,
why does this myth persist? Another way of asking this question is "Who benefits from the perspective of scarcity?" If there
were enough to go around so that all of us could equally pros-
per, how could some of us be seen as better than the rest of us?
To be on top, someone needs to be on the bottom. If everyone
got As, how could I be seen as the smartest person in the class?
Thus, to justify any kind of high status, those who enjoy it find
ways to justify that they have more than the next person of
whatever skills are in question. No one could be on top if everyone were equally deserving. In other words, to maintain
high status, we create the criteria, the yardsticks, that keep us
there.

It's not easy to counteract the assumption of scarcity and
the normal distribution. If I have a "limited" resource to
dispense—say, glowing letters of recommendation—I give it
to those who received As in my classes, rarely reflecting on

what determined the grade in any particular year. My decision-making seminar happened to bring out some brilliant students, and thus there are times they all deserved and got As. After my university spotted this, I was taken to task by the higher-ups. They sent me a printout showing how each student to whom I gave an A did in his or her other classes, revealing that my grade was an outlier. There are pressures against seeing every student as smart in some way. This doesn't mean we should abolish grades or tests. Rather, I object to how we *treat* grades, seeing them as inviolable measures of success.

Of course, some resources are treated as limited. Imagine, for instance, a university department that has three openings for graduate students and fifty applicants. The department must decide who is most worthy based on some predetermined criteria of deservedness. The problem with this is *who* determines the criteria. The people who set the standards are humans, after all, and as with our discussion of rules in chapter 1, different people see things differently. In addition to this inherent flaw in trying to create objective markers, there's another problem: What happens if we have fifty available spots next year? Because we now believe the arbitrary criteria are objective, I believe we would still use the original criteria to select students and would leave some positions unfilled rather than question the criteria.

When we don't recognize the arbitrary nature of the original criteria, we don't seek more mindful solutions. Believing in set criteria makes it easier to make decisions and to believe that the logic that went into creating the standards is time- and circumstance-proof. In other words, because we chose graduate students based on specific criteria in the past, we act as if that must be the optimal way to continue to choose graduate students. If someone, for example, had low grades in college, she or he would probably be rejected outright, but an argument certainly could be made for the person who had abysmal grades and was also the first author on a published paper.

Here's another example: When I was a preteen, my father coached in our town's baseball Little League. Each season, he'd first ask me to hit balls in certain directions to see how well I could control my swing. He hit fly balls to see how well I could catch them in the outfield, and he hit ground balls to me in the infield. My age and baseball talent then imprinted on him a standard by which he'd later evaluate the new crop of boys trying out. Those boys who could do as well as I did could play on the team. I, of course, could not, because back then Little League was just for boys. Though I am amazed in retrospect by the arbitrariness of this convention, I never saw it as odd when it was happening. Girls simply weren't good enough to play. Period.

On another occasion, in an honors high school English class, I chose to write a paper on Edgar Allan Poe. The teacher disparaged me for my choice before even knowing my approach to the topic. To her, there were topics worth writing about and others that were not. I switched to write about Ezra Pound, a decision of which she approved. I gathered that the more ostensibly difficult the poems, the more respect she had for a poet.

I've seen this play out in my work as well. The results of my experiments and studies are often seen as too simple to be true. I maintain that it is hard making things look simple.

Where do we get the idea that complexity and difficulty are more related to quality of thought than simplicity? Consider all of the thought that went into creating Einstein's "simple" formula $E=mc^2$.

Talent, ability, intelligence, and personal characteristics like friendliness and generosity are also generally seen as "normally distributed." We blithely go about our business once we know where we fall on the continuum, never questioning who chose the criteria and how life would be different if other people did the choosing or the same people chose differently.

Musical talent is definitely seen as limited. When my teacher in junior high school had us all choose a song to sing in front of the class, I chose one called "Oh My Papa" and practiced strenuously but with dread. I can carry a tune, I'm told, just not very far. Each student got up in turn. Mine was approaching. The person right before me couldn't carry a tune, either. The teacher was nice to her and reprimanded the class for their groans. I knew I was in trouble; I knew that meant I would take the brunt of her need to critique us. If she were nice to all of us in this way, she wouldn't be able to make the point the drill was implicitly designed to make—to show that musical ability varied widely among us. Unfortunately, I was correct. She made clear that I was not among the talented kids in the class. It wasn't entirely humiliating, but it also wasn't fun. When I compare tonal with atonal music from the East, or consider singers like Leonard Cohen and Bob Dylan, whose poetry makes voice quality less important, I question the criteria being used to identify talent. I'm not alone in this view. David Bowie wrote a song for Bob Dylan that said Dylan's voice was like sand and glue.

The widespread assumption of limited resources is built into our language. One sign of this catches my ear every time I hear it. Say I have a dinner date with a friend and she calls me to say, "I'm almost ready to leave, I just have to take *my* shower." I usually feel like responding, "No take mine." On other occasions, she might tell me that she's having *her* lunch. Many people I've come to know over the years have the same linguistic habit. I wonder if they would still need to proclaim ownership in this way if they had grown up in situations of plentitude. As Tennyson so aptly wrote, "Walls do not a prison make." When you live in a world of perceived scarcity, much time is spent worrying about the scarce resource. In a world of plentitude, there's room for more interesting things to ponder.

JUST TRY HARDER

Limiting the available number of lofty positions is often justified by the hard work that those at the top purportedly had to do to get there. We are invested in the idea that the effort is difficult; trying, via this logic, is inherently unpleasant even if we're pleased if we finally succeed. This view only serves to discourage us from beginning the activity.

Of course, if we find that something is unpleasant to do, we may try to overcome the feeling and do it anyway. Given that the distaste is in our heads and not in the task, thinking differently about it is likely to be more successful. No matter how hard I try not to overeat, not to be stressed, or not to be angry, I am likely to overeat and get even more stressed and angry if I frame my attempts at self-improvement in terms of willful effort. Why can't I make myself go to the gym? Trying harder in the absence of other changes can easily make things worse.

We wouldn't fail so much if we respected our choices more. If something doesn't taste good, why eat it? If you don't like the gym, why not find a more pleasurable form of exercise? Rather than trying to do the thing we hate doing, we can try to find an alternative. If that's not possible—and often it seems it is not—the key is to reframe the thing we hate doing so it is not painful. Almost anything can be made pleasurable if we don't tell ourselves we have to do it. When we make it fun, trying becomes unnecessary. Consider how odd it sounds to *try* to eat something you like eating or *do* something you like doing. If we enjoy pizza or chocolate cake, eating it isn't much of a chore. If we enjoy doing something, it will feel effortless. When we're mindfully engaged, we don't notice the presence or absence of effort.

There is a widespread misconception that effort is something that needs to be minimized. It does appear that way when you are doing something mindlessly or reluctantly. If you are told to wash the dishes, you may slouch and scrub laconically. Heaven forbid you put any real effort into it. If you were asked to describe the task afterward, you might say it was hard. But if you want to surprise someone with clean dishes, you do it fast and with a smile. Effort? What effort?

Being mindful essentially eviscerates the idea of effort. When I play tennis, I objectively expend a lot of effort. But I wouldn't put it in those terms. If you rip open a wrapped and sealed package because there is a gift inside, you wouldn't even think about the concept of effort, even though it might have taken quite a bit of it.

Many years ago, research assistant Sophia Snow and I did an experiment where we had people perform the same task, but for half of them we labeled it work and for the other half we labeled it play.[1] Despite the fact that the task was rating cartoons, which might seem inherently fun, those who saw it as work didn't enjoy it; their minds wandered, and they were pleased when the experimental session was over. Those who saw it as "play," in contrast, enjoyed the task. Furthermore, we found that those who had been asked to play at rating cartoons also felt they were being productive. Those who had been asked to do the "work" of rating the same cartoons felt they were less so. Examples of this abound: Tom Sawyer saw painting the fence as work; his friends didn't. Doing one's own dishes isn't fun but doing a friend's dishes after a meal may be. The important takeaway here is to remember that tasks are neither universally considered fun nor arduous. It depends on how we approach them.

Many companies try to make work seem more fun to encourage productivity. For example, Google has Ping-Pong tables in their offices, and kitchenettes stocked with organic and delicious snacks. By most accounts, this kind of incentivizing may work in the short term and induce people to do something they don't find enticing. But rather than a "spoonful of sugar to help the medicine go down," it is far better to make the medicine taste better. I believe that virtually any activity can be authentically fun. Adding something to work to make it palatable only reinforces the idea that it is inherently distasteful.

But if everyone enjoyed what they were doing and did it relatively effortlessly and well, how would the people at the top maintain their positions? Scarcity requires suffering for some of us. Does being healthy need to be effortful?

SORTING WINNERS AND LOSERS

One of the most pernicious consequences of the scarcity mindset is that it leads us to sort people into winners and losers, haves and have-nots. Some people are nicer or less nice, or more or less talented, and so more or less deserving of our limited resources.

The need for sorting winners and losers begins early. When I was in high school, I saw a girl crying at the gym because she had not been asked to join a popular sorority. Because my sister had been a member, I had been deemed a "legacy" and allowed to join. I felt bad about this unfairness, so I got some of the more popular girls in school together at my house where we all decided to quit the sorority. Joking around, we decided to call ourselves the Elites. Twenty some odd years later, I made contact with an old friend from high school who hadn't been there the day we quit the sorority. She told me how she had suffered by not being one of the Elites. As they say, life is complicated.

As a graduate student in psychology at Yale, I worked at the Yale Psycho-Educational Clinic. The patients paid for their therapy and often traveled some distance to get there, which was a good indication that they were motivated to change their behavior. Too often, they still failed to change. I had been taught that if people were motivated to change and showed that they knew what needed to be done, they would do it, so I was frustrated by those who got stuck. I wanted to tell them to "just do it," but I also knew that wouldn't be considered good therapy. Then I realized that, despite what they said, these patients might actually value the very behaviors they said they wanted to change.

One of my Harvard undergraduates, Loralyn Thompson, and I decided to test this.[2] We gave people a sheet of paper that had on it about one hundred behavior descriptors and asked participants to circle those things they wanted to change but had been unable to do so. On the reverse side of the sheet, in a random order, were the positive versions of each of these negative behavior characteristics. Now their task was to circle those things they value about themselves. Thus, one side had listed things such as inconsistent, impulsive, gullible, inflexible, and grim, while on the reverse side it listed flexible, spontaneous, trusting, stable, and serious. Sure enough, most of the very things that people tried unsuccessfully to change were the things they actually valued about themselves when cast in a positive light.

When I look back at different events in my life, given this understanding, they make sense to me. One summer when I was around twelve, I befriended an unpopular girl at camp because I felt sorry for her. I spent a good deal of time with her and hoped others would follow suit. They didn't. Eventually I backed off from this new friendship a bit, after having given her what I thought was much generosity. She saw it differently and felt betrayed by my abandoning her rather than grateful for our time together. While I still think I was doing something nice, now I realize that from her perspective I was being condescending, not generous.

Many people believe the way to be nonjudgmental is to be more accepting of others and to accept their "weaknesses." My view is quite different. I believe that recognizing the sense to someone else's behavior is a path to being nonjudgmental. If I question someone's behavior, but then ask what that person was intending, the behavior virtually always seems to make sense, even if I disagree with their result. I don't judge them harshly or think they should change unless they want to. I could stop being gullible, for example, but since I value being trusting I choose not to.

Consider bullying. For many people, bullies are bad actors who prey on those less powerful. They should be scorned and punished when possible. The stereotype of what people experience when bullied is that the bully is strong, which is why they make us feel weak and scared. But what is happening from the bully's perspective? I see the bully as someone who feels deeply insecure—the only way he knows to feel good about himself is to pick on someone else. If we viewed the bully in this light, we might be more likely to feel sorry for him than afraid. If we're not afraid, there is no motivation for him to bully us.

This was my response when I learned someone I cared about had defrauded me out of a huge sum of money. Even though I felt betrayed, my most overwhelming emotion was feeling sorry for him.

SOMEONE ELSE'S SHOES: THE PROBLEM WITH
PERSPECTIVE TAKING

The adage that we should not judge another person until
we've walked a mile in their shoes would benefit from more
thought. Consider the story of the Prince and the Pauper.[3] The
Prince wants to find out what it's like to be a pauper and so
goes out from the kingdom donning clothes befitting an out-
cast. As I remember the story, living among the poor, he thinks
he learns firsthand what life is like for those far less fortunate
than he. Does the prince now have the perspective of a pauper? With this new wisdom, can he rule more justly? To my
mind, the answer is no.

For me, the worst thing about being a pauper would probably be not knowing if I was ever going to have enough food
to eat or to be safe. These are things that the prince, even when
he is playing the pauper, can count on. All he has to do is stop
trying to take the pauper's perspective and go back to being
princely again. The pauper does not have the luxury of this
choice.

Consider it this way. The advice we're too often given is
that perspective is solely the result of being exposed to the
same information given in the same way. If this were so, then
all we have to do to understand how someone else might feel
is to see the information "from their perspective." But if you
literally walked in my shoes, wouldn't your feet mold the
leather in ways different from mine? I'm used to the way my
feet feel and so over time, I've grown sensitive to some things
and numb to others. To these matters you are oblivious. If the

way we understand and feel about information is the cumulative result of our life's experience, then, having lived my life and not yours, I cannot really know how you feel.

What then is to be learned from walking in another's moccasins? Rather than believe that now, after presumably taking the other's perspective, we really know what it feels like to be another, the walk could reveal how much we *didn't* know before. If we did this often enough, we'd be more likely to ask people what they want and need, and trust their answers rather than assume we know.

In relationships, oddly enough given the fact that similar tastes may have brought us together, we tend to focus on our differences. One of us will always be better than the other at whatever we're considering because no two people are exactly equal with respect to anything. Although both of us may be more neat than sloppy, and reasonably good at handling money, necessarily, one of us will be a little neater, or a little better at handling money.

These differences often become magnified and frozen in our minds—one becomes a slob, and one becomes someone who has trouble managing money. To make the point more personal, my spouse and I both have good memories. Nevertheless, she is sure her memory is better than mine. She'll ask me about some event, and I may have no idea what she is referring to. When we had the experience in the first place, we found different things interesting about it and so in some ways we experienced different events. Thus, the way she recalls "her" event may be entirely different from the way I recall "mine." To her, however, I could appear forgetful. Another perspective would see a difference, not a deficit.

It's interesting to ask how much of the presumed memory loss attributed to the old is a result of this difference in perspective. If you were testing memory with words like "mahjong" and "pinochle" versus "Game Boy" and "Warcraft," my guess is that senior citizens would remember more about the former since those were the common games of their youth, and young adults the latter. In other words, much of what is taken as memory loss is a difference in values, not memory. If I don't learn it in the first place because I don't care, when I later don't know it, it's not because I forgot it—it's because I never learned it. In a world that presumes limited personal abilities, naïve realism prevails—that there is but one way to understand events.

In his charming book *Exercises in Style*, Raymond Queneau retells a simple story about two men meeting on a bus from different perspectives.[4] You might think that since there are two people involved in the encounter there would be only two perspectives, but Queneau tells the tale from ninety-nine different perspectives. While I'm not suggesting we try to see situations in so many ways, realizing it is possible allows us to see there is not a single reality shared by us all.

Even the smartest among us can fall into the trap of seeing from a single perspective. Robert Abelson, my mentor at Yale, and I were going to do a study on the perception of "crazy." We never got past trying to create the stimuli that would signal crazy for the study. He would say, "A woman puts a candy wrapper in the refrigerator." I would say, "That's not crazy. She's trying to remind herself that she's already consumed enough calories for the day when she reaches for a refrigerated dessert." He would say a man stays awake into the wee hours of the morning obsessing over something. I would say he's not obsessing, he's problem-solving and not all problems have quick solutions. This went on and on and on.

Eventually my implicit belief became an explicit thesis: Behavior makes sense from the actor's perspective or else she or he wouldn't have done it. Of all that I've written in the course of my career, this may be the most important insight to me. In a psychological review paper, Mihnea Moldoveanu and I showed how several different interpretations of the same results in behavioral decision theory and cognitive psychology are all well supported by the "facts" if we consider multiple perspectives.[5] People seen by psychologists as "weakly conforming" might be better understood as helping social interactions to unfold more seamlessly; those of us seen as gullible may be better understood as trusting, and so on. Although the scarcity mindset leads us to see our differences as deficits, it doesn't have to be this way.

How can we rise above this scarcity mindset? I think we can learn from some research I did on eyesight, which also reveals how a belief in scarcity is related to health problems. In particular, the research is a reminder that many of the physical limitations we assume are inevitable with age are largely the products of our mindset, and not our body.

In one experiment, we recruited students from MIT's ROTC program. After testing the students using a standard vision test, we asked them to "become pilots" by using a flight simulator.[6] Because Air Force pilots are believed to have better eyesight—20/20 vision is a requirement—we hypothesized that the students would show improved vision while playing the part of pilots in the simulator. (We even had them wear pilot uniforms to enhance their sense of role-playing.) Sure enough, by asking them to read tiny numbers and letters while using the simulator, we were able to show that 40 percent of the "pilots," but none of the control participants, displayed improved vision. Their new mindset eliminated their physical limitation; the mind "improved," and thus so did the body.

We then replicated these results with a larger sample of students. Instead of asking them to pretend to be pilots, we asked them to do jumping jacks for a few minutes in order to prime an "athletic" mindset. Once again, about a third of people in the athletic frame of mind showed enhanced vision. In another experiment, we inverted the standard eye chart, so that the letters became larger, not smaller, as one read down. Again, this led to improved performance because we changed people's expectations. People believed they would be able to see the letters as you go down the chart, and so they did see the letters they wouldn't "normally" be able to identify. The moral, of course, is that no such normal exists. We can see more than we think.

Too often, we let our assumptions about scarcity dictate our behavior and health. We become hard on ourselves and judgmental of others. We assume we can't get stronger or smarter or improve our eyesight since some of us are just destined to be less than others. We assume stress is a necessary evil. My hope is that we can learn to see past the myth of scarcity and experience a world of enhanced possibility.

When 3M failed to make a glue that adheres, it could have discarded the chemical concoction as a failure. Instead, it mindfully created the Post-it Note, a product whose essence depends on its *inability* to adhere well. This created a brand-new resource and office products category. Once we realize that most things can serve multiple purposes rather than the single original purpose for which it was intended, new resources are constantly coming into being.

If we adopt new mindsets, and learn to look past the myth of scarcity, we can find new opportunities in our changing bodies.

CHAPTER 4

Why Decide?

Once you make a decision, the universe
conspires to make it happen.
Attributed to RALPH WALDO EMERSON

There are probably few things as stressful as having to make a difficult decision. And every time we're faced with these decisions, our bodies suffer. When I began to look for a teaching position in 1974, I went for several taxing job interviews. I was interested in a job at Harvard, but I decided not to pursue it because at the time they didn't tenure junior faculty. I was excited when I was offered a position at Carnegie Mellon, all the more so because when Carnegie's famed decision theorist—and Nobel Prize winner—Herb Simon found out it was my birthday, he and a colleague called me to sing "Happy Birthday" over the phone. But I was also offered a job at the Graduate Center of the City University of New York, my home city. I clearly had great options, but deciding which job to accept felt like a decision of monumental importance: I was scared I would make the wrong decision and destroy my future life.

When I was visiting Carnegie Mellon we talked a lot about research and psychology in general, but at CUNY we talked a lot about food—and about the arts and politics, not research findings. What did these differences suggest? Which school would be a better fit? What decision should I have made?

This was an important life choice, and I approached it quite seriously. I gathered lots of information about each school. I worried about the choice and probably lost some sleep in the process. One of my professors at Yale, Irving Janis, taught that the best way to make a decision was to write out the options and the advantages and disadvantages for each (for him it was as if the list was finite) and then weigh them based on importance (for him as if that was stable). I followed his recommendation, and CUNY kept coming up short. As a born and bred New Yorker, the CUNY job really appealed to me in a very personal way, so I kept recalibrating my lists, changing the relative "weights" of advantages and disadvantages to make it come out on top on paper. Then I accepted that offer and was happy teaching there for several years.

Was this the right decision? What would my life be like now if I had started my teaching career at Carnegie Mellon? There's no way of knowing. There's no way of finding out.

One summer after I had joined the Graduate Center, however, CUNY was facing financial problems, and faculty paychecks were delayed. I was concerned enough that I decided to find out what other jobs might be available, just in case. I saw a job posted for a clinical psychologist at the Graduate School of Education at Harvard. I wasn't really qualified, but I applied anyway. The faculty on the search committee at the School of Education recognized that I wasn't an appropriate candidate for their position but rather than just putting my application aside, they surprisingly forwarded it to Brendan Maher, then chair of the psychology department in Harvard College. I would not have predicted this.

He was interested and after the requisite interviews, Brendan called to offer me a position in the psychology department. I was flattered, but I told him that I knew Harvard didn't tenure junior faculty so was not inclined to accept the offer. In response, he explained that while it was true Harvard hadn't yet tenured junior faculty, that was not a policy, and tenure was likely in the cards for me.

Since I could no longer come up with a list of serious disadvantages, I was elated, and packed for Cambridge. Should I have considered more options and done a cost-benefit analysis? What would that have bought me? Some decisions, like this one, seem clear and easy and obvious. While I couldn't predict the outcome, it was an exciting opportunity.

DECISION SYSTEMS

In the 1990s, the dominant view of decision-making among psychologists was in line with Irv Janis's logical list comparison.[1] Successful decisions were thought to be made by calculating the probable costs and benefits for each of the considered alternatives. Essentially psychologists were just adopting the rational agent model from economics. To it they then added subjective experience—the idea that a benefit for one person could be irrelevant for another. Formally, this is called subjective expected utility theory.

Obviously, I didn't make my decision in this way, so it's not surprising that my decision-making theory was completely at odds with this view. Moreover, I didn't think people in general did tedious cost-benefit analyses to make their decisions. But before I share my ideas about how we do and should make decisions, it's important to understand how the field has progressed.

In recent years, decision-making theorizing has evolved to include two models of how people make decisions. Nobel prize winner Daniel Kahneman coined the terms "system 1" and "system 2" thinking to describe these two basic paths.[2] System 1 is mindless decision-making. It is fast, driven by instinct and prior learning, and often relies on mental shortcuts or heuristics. For example, you see a sign for Burger King and make an unplanned turn off the highway for french fries, or you happily respond to a call from a friend who has an extra ticket to see your favorite singer, or you put on your favorite outfit for a job interview without considering other possibilities. In these instances, we are not consciously doing any cost-benefit analysis; we are just acting intuitively.

Alternatively, in Kahneman's system 2 decision-making system, we take the time and effort to reflect on our options. Should I remain in my current job? Or accept a new offer? Which house should I buy? In these decisions we compare options, look for costs and benefits, and, often, get stressed over what to do. At first glance, system 2 may seem mindful.

While system 1 and system 2 bear clear similarities to mindlessness and mindfulness, in my view those resemblances are illusory, and both of these modes of decision-making are or can be flawed. Unless we want to call everything a decision, system 1 "decisions" are mindless and as such are not really decisions at all, any more than I "decide" which letter to hit on the keyboard when typing my name. To my mind, we are not making a decision if we are unaware at the time of other actions we might consider taking. Being mindless, we go forward oblivious to opportunities in front of us or to ways of averting dangers not yet arisen.

To me, system 2 can also be mindless, and this is where I have diverged from the consensus of some of my peers. System 2 thinking is not inherently mindful precisely because it *is* inherently effortful. Consider adding 372 and 26. Although not a decision, per se, it'll help make the point. While not very difficult, it requires some effort for most of us. The effort comes from applying information we learned by rote memorization to arrive at an answer. In this example, to arrive at the answer we first add 2 plus 6, which for most of us is always 8. As such, it is mindless. Mindfulness is defined as actively noticing novelty or considering new alternatives. We typically don't consider alternatives when doing arithmetic.

I'm not sure how to mindfully add 372 and 26, but that doesn't mean arithmetic can't be done mindfully. For example, when I ask, "How much is 1 + 1?," people mindlessly respond "2." They could instead realize that it depends on what is being added. If you add one pile of laundry to another pile of laundry, you still have one pile of laundry. If we've individually added 372 pieces of laundry to a pile, it becomes more effortful as the task continues, but there is nothing new to the process, so it is not mindful. Now, if we still have patience, let's individually add 26 more pieces of laundry. The answer is still one pile. Mindfulness is not effortful in the traditional way we think of effort. What is effortful is mindlessly trying to pay attention to something without recognizing anything new about it. It takes effort to shop for a gift for someone you don't really like, and it takes effort to buy something for someone you love. But they are different. The first one is mindless and exhausting as we keep the thought of having to find something in our minds. The second is often mindful, exhilarating, and energizing. We tend, however, to conflate the two. As a result, we are too often oblivious to how energizing mindful effort can be.

System 2 cost-benefit analyses are also mindless because we lock in what is a cost and what is a benefit based on conditions from an earlier time. Any cost can also be a benefit if viewed differently. At present, things may be quite different for us but we're blind to those differences unless we mindfully consider them. The perfect house you thought you always wanted to buy may no longer suit you if you reconsidered it now. The job that once fit your skills now seems dreary.

Consider being offered the chance to buy your friend's summer cottage that you have always coveted. Ten years ago, when your friend first bought it, you were envious because it was on the water and had great views. But those memories may cloud your current decision, even if you think you recognize that it is less valuable because it does not have the latest energy-saving appliances, or that it is vulnerable to environmental changes that have eroded the shoreline. Even if you think you can calculate how much it is worth on the current market compared to other nearby properties, and think how much you will enjoy sitting on the deck, you can't predict or know if the water will become so warm that it will destroy the shellfish, or if the beach will disappear, or if people who play loud music all night will purchase the house next door. But, if we mindlessly ignore most of this, and simply look at the current price of the house compared to others in the neighborhood, our system 2 decision will tell us to buy it. Thus, most system 2 decisions are mindless.

INFINITE REGRESS

Here's where my view starts to diverge even more. As with the cottage above, when people weigh costs and the benefits to make a decision, there's no end to potentially relevant information and no way of knowing the limits of what you could or should consider. Take a cost-benefit analysis of a cookie. The costs and the benefits are all in your head and not in the cookie. Costs and benefits incorporate your expectations and interpretations. The cookie's sugar, for instance, might be bad for your teeth. On the other hand, its sweetness is satisfying, which leads you to produce more ptyalin, an enzyme present in saliva that helps us digest starches, which is actually good for your teeth. So how do you decide?

In *Hamlet*, Shakespeare shows us that overthinking can be dangerous. Hamlet spends more time on thought than taking action. He wants to avenge his father's death and obsesses over it for almost the entire play. And it's not just in literature. Mathematician and business strategist Igor Ansoff shows us the same problem in business decisions. But most of us experience this in mundane situations almost every day.[3] Writing about shopping for a pair of jeans, psychologist Barry Schwartz describes his "analysis paralysis" to describe the nearly universal phenomenon of believing that there is a single correct decision and if we just search hard enough, we'll find it.[4] The salesperson asked Schwartz if he wanted slim fit, relaxed fit, baggy, or extra baggy. Then she asked about his preference for the wash: She wanted to know if he wanted stonewashed, acid-washed, or distressed. By the time he had to decide if he wanted button or zipper fly he realized that having choices felt good until there was too much to decide.

Instead of trying to make the best choice, Schwartz suggests we should employ a concept first described by Carnegie Melon's Herb Simon: satisfice.[5] That is, make a choice that is good enough. Simon, Schwartz, and probably most other people believe there are still objectively better and worse choices, but the process of finding them is too costly to engage.

I don't think that more information, more time, and more calculations are better. Rather than all this information improving our decisions, it can result in dissatisfaction and almost crippling anxiety. After all, working memory is not unlimited, and new information can be distracting.

Moreover, in general, most people don't consider a great deal of information before making a decision. Relevant to this is a study psychologist Chuck Kiesler conducted in the late sixties in which people were given either two or four alternatives of candy bars from which to choose.[6] One might imagine that with more choices, people would spend more time making the decision. In fact, he found the opposite: The more choices, the faster they chose. And in a later series of studies,

Barry Schwartz and his colleagues found that considering many options and taking in a good deal of information results in a decrease in happiness, self-esteem, satisfaction with one's life, and optimism. It was also correlated with an increase in depression, perfectionism, and regret. Similar to Kiesler before her, psychologist Sheena Iyengar offered people jams to taste and then purchase. Some participants were given six flavors to taste, while others could taste twenty-four different varieties.[7] None of the people who tasted twenty-four jams chose to buy any of them while a number of the people who tried six flavors made a purchase. Iyengar found the same was true for important decisions like retirement savings. When 401(k) plans offered the choice of one or two funds, many more people participated than when plans offered many funds from which to choose.

Similarly, branding expert Martin Lindstrom conducted an experiment in which employees at a large bookstore chain removed all but one of the store's display tables, so that instead of hundreds of titles, only ten books were on display.[8] Sales increased. All of these examples show that having more options to choose from is not better.

MAKING THE DECISION RIGHT

Too often, we divide the world into mindless dichotomies. You either have control or you don't. But the real question is: Control over what? And from whose perspective?

This is especially true when it comes to medical decisions. For the vast majority, if not all, of such decisions, the outcomes are probabilistic and full of uncertainty. Which treatment should you choose? The doctor will typically frame the alternatives in terms of potential outcomes.

Take the question of knee surgery, a common dilemma among my friends. On the one hand, maybe you shouldn't get surgery because the injury might resolve on its own and surgery is always risky. On the other hand, it might get worse and require even more extensive surgery if you wait. Of course, if you delay the surgery, a better procedure might be invented. But if you do it now you can get back to your regular exercise schedule. And so on. If you're so inclined, you can always check the empirical literature, but that's usually just as confusing.

So how should we make decisions? We should begin by recognizing our limitations; the human brain is not an omnipotent supercomputer. Moreover, even if it were, there's the "problem" that every cost is also a benefit from a different perspective. As a result, when making decisions in uncertainty, more information, time, and calculations are not better. In fact, taking too much information into account can backfire, leading people to overthink the problem and choke. Sian Beilock and Thomas Carr's work shows this at work in an educational setting.[9] If we are anxious about a math problem, we consider too many possibilities, which can consume our scarce working memory and keep us from solving the problem at hand. We're so worried about getting it right that we get it wrong.

Imagine deciding whether to buy a house. What states, cities, or neighborhoods to consider? How much can you really afford to pay? To answer this question, we might need to know what the economy will look like in five years; whether the stock market will grow or shrink; whether our jobs will remain secure; whether unexpected expenses will occur; whether we'll remain married and continue to need a house; whether we'll continue to want the costs of home ownership, and so on. The list is almost endless, and each of the pieces of information above have their own inherent uncertainties and risks.

This doesn't mean we should buy a house at random, or not buy a house at all. Instead, I would argue for a very different approach. Rather than recommending endless analysis, my experience and research suggest taking a limited amount of information available at the time and going ahead and choosing an option. Then, rather than worry about whether the decision was right, we should try to *make it work.* Look at any advantages that accrue from whatever happens, and then play it as the "right decision." That is, *don't try to make the right decision, make the decision right.* In this case, once you have chosen a house to buy, you can "make the decision right" by starting to build investments in your neighborhood—registering your kids in local schools, knocking on doors to meet your neighbors, and joining the local gym—and by making your new home warm and inviting by finding a table and chairs to fit in your new kitchen, helping your daughter set up the Wi-Fi for her computer in her bedroom, and finding the local Little League for your son.

The same applies to medical plans. That is, *don't try to make the right decision, make the decision right by enrolling in a local gym or signing up for physical therapy after knee surgery.* We can never be sure our knee wouldn't heal on its own or with just a consistent practice of yoga, or whether some new magical drug would soon be coming to market. We can never be sure the surgery will be successful. On the other hand, the surgery could be successful and we finally could be pain free post-surgery. Regardless of whether you have the surgery, the next step is basically the same: Do all that you can to regain the pain-free life you're seeking. Satisficing suggests there is a correct answer but it's too hard to figure out. My view is that there is no correct decision independent of the decider making it right.

Many years ago, I was talking to my friend the economist and Nobel laureate Thomas Schelling about my decision theory. He told me he came to basically the same conclusion after he went to buy a microwave oven. Having never had a microwave, he had no idea how he'd use it. Would he want a special button for popcorn or cooking salmon? Or would he just use it to reheat his coffee? Not being able to know in advance, he concluded that the best decision was just to buy one of them and see if he needed more or fewer options. Instead of obsessing over the alternatives, he just made a choice and then tried to make the best of it. If nothing else, he'd learn from his mistakes. I added that even if he decided to buy his next one with fewer features because they went unused, it still would be a blind decision because he could not know how his life might change. After all, perhaps his wife or child would learn much more about microwaves at a friend's house and now have use for the extra features.

Watching a friend who could never make up her mind and was ambivalent about almost everything helped me understand something novel about decision-making—that there is no natural endpoint to the amount of information we can consider for any decision. I was often frustrated when we planned to go out to dinner and she spent so much time trying to decide where to go and what to order. The underlying problem was my friend's belief that there was a single right decision. I think this is the reason for all ambivalence. While it is easy to see that there is no right decision when deciding about the choice of a restaurant (or which blue jeans to buy, as in the above example), it turns out to be true in virtually all cases. Importantly, there is no limit to the amount of information or to the number of alternative actions we could take.

Imagine, for example, receiving a tax refund of $3,000. What do you do with the money? Put it all in the bank? Buy stocks and if so, which ones? Put some of it in the bank and invest the rest and if so, how much for each? Spend some of the money and put the rest in the bank, but spend it on what, and set aside how much? And so on and so on. Not only is the list of options virtually endless, the possible and reasonable pros and cons of any of these alternatives are also endless. When we think of consequences for each alternative, we are limited only by our willingness and stamina to go through the process and generate possibilities.

That is not a realistic way to make decisions.

NO WRONG DECISION

I come at decision-making another way. I'm equally in favor of making decisions by factoring in the information available at the time or by ignoring it. But then, once we choose an option, I suggest that we make it work rather than worrying about whether the decision was right. We can play any choice as the right decision by looking at any advantages that accrue. Again, that is, *don't try to make the right decision, make the decision right.*

Sounds crazy, right? To test whether this is a reasonable strategy, I asked students in my decision seminar to spend the week until our next class saying yes to all requests. Want to go out for Italian food? Yes. Want to see that new movie? Yes. Want to take a walk in the rain? Yes. Unless someone asked them to do something they felt was wrong or dangerous, they would say yes without taking time to decide. The majority of students reported back that the week had gone better than they expected. They didn't struggle with any decision. There was no stress. When they hesitated, not knowing what to do, they remembered that I had given them permission—indeed, a directive—to just say "yes."

Another year I asked my students to make all of their decisions for a week in an arbitrary way. I told them to use a rule for each decision that had no relevance for that particular decision. I suggested, for instance, that they always choose the first alternative that came to mind or the last. Whether the decisions were significant or not, these students also reported back that already having decided to simply respond according to the arbitrary rule had made their week less stressful as well.

The next year, I asked the students to spend the week seeing every little task as a decision to be made. Rather than just put on shoes, for example, make "Should I put on shoes?" a decision. And then the choice of *which* shoes another decision. And the choice of when to put them on a decision. And so on.

You might think that these students had a totally different experience than the ones whose decisions were predetermined, but instead many of them felt that living this way was helpful and even kind of fun. This suggests that when you have many decisions to make, you can better tolerate getting some of them "wrong." It's like the difference between a test that has only one question on it and a test made up of one hundred questions. There's a lot of pressure on getting the one question "right."

The problem with current views of decision-making is that we tend to get stressed not only by consequential decisions but also by inconsequential ones. I myself have been stymied by whether to buy a Milky Way or a Snickers. Decide or randomly choose? Both strategies seem to work regardless of the importance of the decision. We're fine if we make decisions and we're fine if we don't—at least as long as we feel we have permission not to do so.

There's a standard "puzzle" in decision theory involving irrelevant alternatives that illustrates the way we often make decisions. If you go to a big-box store, you'll see they sell one huge and expensive TV that's rarely purchased. But the presence of that TV makes people view the second-most expensive TV as a bargain. Most analyses of this phenomenon conclude that people are irrational by being influenced by an irrelevant option and implicitly think there is a correct decision. Those researchers, however, fail to follow the people home. Once the TV is in the house, the irrelevant alternative is gone. Do people then "come to their senses" and return the TV? No, what matters is that they make their decision right. They enjoy their purchase. If they had gone to a different store that didn't offer the irrelevant expensive alternative, they may have purchased a different TV, and then been happy with that decision as well; that is, they will have made *that* decision right.

WHEN DECISIONS MATTER

Don't people in positions of power need to do cost-benefit analyses to arrive at just and equitable decisions? Consider an interesting study on judicial decision-making by Shai Danziger, now at Tel Aviv University, and his colleagues.[10] They looked at parole decisions as a function of food breaks the judges take. Favorable decisions reliably drop from 65 percent to zero before a food break and increase back to 65 percent after. The findings at first are amusing, but given the implications for anyone appearing before a judge for possible parole, they become frightening. We assume that judicial rulings are based on an enormous amount of legal knowledge and precedents. Instead, they found that the decisions made by experienced judges were instead most influenced by how hungry the judges were.

Psychologists argue persuasively that not infrequently—but paradoxically—reasoning can lead to bad decisions. They maintain that we make our decisions based on the alternative that's easiest to justify to other people, rather than after a search for a better answer. Moreover, often, we care more about not looking stupid than choosing the best alternative. And, actually, that's fine since there is no objectively right decision.

When I had to decide whether to get into the Jeep in the Virgin Islands or wait for a bus that might never come, I neither did a cost-benefit analysis nor worried about how to justify my decision to others. All I knew was that I was afraid to continue waiting so I got into the Jeep. Some of the best decisions are made without any justification at all. Indeed, justifications are not expected in emergencies. The nature of an emergency is that there is no time for an elaborate search for alternatives, cost-benefit analyses, and so forth. Nevertheless, decisions are made, actions are taken.

Consumer behavior tells the same story. Many buyers decide on their purchases in under three seconds. Indeed, when I'm at a restaurant and open the menu and see they have soft-shell crabs, I probably come in under two seconds. Some people, however, can't seem to cross the goal line in making a decision—whether about which coat to buy or what to eat. In the first instance, the quick deciders don't take enough time to do a cost-benefit analysis. For the "can't make a decision" group, even if they do the calculations, it doesn't seem to help.

It seems that although people may think they should look at as much information as possible, they usually don't. This is true even for people whose jobs are mostly about making decisions. Iyengar found that CEOs take less than nine minutes to make 50 percent of their decisions. Thus, it's unlikely that they typically do an extensive cost-benefit analysis.

Once a decision is made, we can never know for sure what would have happened if another option had been kept in play. Consider the Las Vegas Sands casino, the Royal Caribbean cruise line, and Micron Technology. These are businesses that respectively lost more than a billion dollars over two years after years of success. You might have argued it would have been reasonable for them to have called it quits after the first year to prevent further losses. But each company decided to stay in business and went on to enjoy considerable growth. I'm not advocating that we never change course. I'm saying that we can't know whether one decision is, or was, necessarily better than another. We can't know what the road not taken would have been like. It could have been better, worse, or not different at all.

Psychologists also take as a given that the consequences of decisions are either good or bad. Important work on what's known as prospect theory shows that, for many people, the hurt from losses outweighs the pleasure from gains, and the way a decision is framed will affect how they make their choice.[11] For example, people may decide to have surgery when it is described as 90 percent likely to be successful, but to avoid it if it is presented as 10 percent likely to be unsuccessful. Although objectively the two choices are the same, the emotions they evoke are very different.

Neurobiologist Antonio Damasio made the field take notice of the effects of emotions on our decisions. Since Plato, the view had been that we need to control our passions.[12] For Damasio, our emotions don't cloud our decisions but rather are and should be critical for decision-making. Because emotions mark things as good, bad, or neutral and we unconsciously build up memories of these feelings, they can then provide a lift when we need to make a decision.

Damasio came to this view primarily as a result of his experience with patients. Those with lesions in the orbitofrontal cortex, which is involved in decision-making, were unable to make a decision. They had no problem doing cost-benefit analyses, but every time they would identify a cost, they would recognize a new benefit. Damasio discovered that his patients were missing the emotional memory that would make something about a decision feel good, bad, or indifferent and help them to make a choice. As a result, they could spend hours with the simplest decision.

My position is different from that of Damasio and other decision theorists who explicitly or implicitly take as a given that consequences are good, bad, or indifferent. Even though they all would acknowledge that what is good for one person may not be good for another and that all of the bad alternatives probably have some good in them and vice versa, they rely on being able to define any given outcome as essentially good or bad. For me, it is not that there are, say, six bad aspects of something and three good aspects, making it essentially bad. My reasoning tells me that each and every aspect is simultaneously good or bad depending on how we frame it. If I asked, "Do you want to go out with my friend John, who is inconsistent and changes his mind a lot?" you'd probably say no, why bother? If instead I had asked you, "Do you want to meet my friend John, who is very flexible in his views?" you might have said yes. Yet inconsistent and cognitively flexible are two ways of describing the same thing.

THE UNRELIABILITY OF PROBABILITY

Probabilities depend on the particular ways we understand something—change the understanding and the probability changes. It might seem obvious that if I flirt with someone, my spouse will probably get angry. But what constitutes "flirting"? What constitutes "getting angry"?

Evaluating past decisions can also go on indefinitely. When we look back at our decisions, we could see them as successful or unsuccessful, depending on which information we call up to consider. It was a good thing we didn't go to that new restaurant, since I surely would have eaten too much. Or it's too bad we didn't go to that new restaurant because it would have been a wonderful experience. We can confirm whatever judgment we choose. You ask me to do something for you. I see you as someone needy, so I may say yes. Or I see you as someone bossy, so I may say no. Because we can change the meaning of anything that happened, most of us can and do justify our decisions. Sadly, though, some of us look for how we decided wrongly. We can prove either case to ourselves. There is no correct decision waiting to be made.

Certainly, some decisions have a greater impact on our lives than others. Deciding which film to see is different from deciding which job to take, whom to marry, or whether to get an operation. Despite the difference in gravity, however, the decision-making process is virtually the same. There are, in theory, an enormous number of consequences we could consider, and each one can be seen as positive or negative. Each new possibility we uncover could change our decision, and there's no rulebook telling us how much information we should consider in the first place. Say that all the available information says you should buy a certain house, but then you come across some news about a highway being built a block away. You decide not to buy the house. Then you find out the city is planning on paying handsomely for houses on the block and you change your mind again. There is no natural endpoint to the potentially relevant information that could be gathered.

Moreover, if every positive can also be viewed as a negative, adding them up as in a cost-benefit analysis will not tell us what the decision should be. (One benefit minus one cost = 0.)

Let's look more closely at "satisficing," Herb Simon's term for a good way to make decisions.[13] He considers using just enough information to make a decision rather than worry about all the potential pieces of information out there. But even if we consider just enough data points to make an informed decision, this strategy still implies that there are better and worse decisions, and more information is better than less. I don't think so. Consider making a decision about taking vitamins. Let's say we consult ten people and they all say it's important to take them. That's 100 percent—pretty convincing. If we ask one hundred people and they all agree, then it would seem even more convincing since it's ten times the amount of information. But we don't know if we asked another hundred or thousand if they would say the same thing. Furthermore, every piece of new information out there could potentially change our minds. Imagine that the one hundred and first person we asked said that their spouse took vitamins not knowing that she was allergic to them and had a crippling reaction as a result.

Moreover, if we were to look closely at each piece of information, we would find many differences behind them. If one hundred people say they've had a good experience with vitamins, how many are taking them every day or just once in a while; how many are shading the truth; for how many is the belief in vitamins a placebo giving them a good experience; and what do they mean by a good experience, anyway?

Health-related decisions can feel especially fraught because we hope for certainty. A doctor told my friend Judy that he had found a mass that might be breast cancer. The doctor recommended a lumpectomy to remove it, suggesting that it would relieve her of worry. While she went ahead and scheduled that surgery, she also decided to get another opinion.

The second doctor asked Judy if she was an Ashkenazi Jew, since there is a genetic predisposition to breast cancer among people with that heritage. When she said yes, the doctor recommended genetic testing but added that there was no point in having genetic testing unless Judy was prepared to consider a double mastectomy if the test revealed she had the gene for breast cancer. Judy told me she was "freaking out" because she was being asked if she was willing to consider a double mastectomy in advance of any diagnosis. At that point, she was totally overwhelmed and asked for my advice.

I said that if that had happened to me, since they weren't sure it was cancer in the first place, I would probably do nothing and have the lump tested every couple of months. And, even if I had the mutant gene, I certainly wouldn't have the double mastectomy because there was only a greater possibility—not a certainty—of developing breast cancer. But that didn't mean she shouldn't. It would depend on how well or poorly she was able to deal with potential stress. It turned out that, for her, the stress of not knowing if the tissue was cancerous was most important. She didn't want to wait for more mammograms. She decided to go ahead with the lumpectomy as the first course of action. But then she found the doctor had scheduled it for the following week—during the Jewish holidays. I wondered out loud to her whether, since she didn't even know whether the lump was cancerous, she might delay that surgery for a month? She breathed a sigh of relief and called the doctor back, and he assured her there was no rush and no crisis and she could take some time to have the lumpectomy. With the pressure removed, she enjoyed the holidays.

She then had the lumpectomy and, fortunately, the growth turned out to be benign. With the stress and pressure removed, she was able to dismiss the need for genetic testing.

Was that the right decision? For her, the pressure to have genetic testing, and to say that she would agree, in advance, to consider a double mastectomy, created so much anxiety that she couldn't think clearly. In the end, resisting that pressure, and heeding my reminder that she didn't even know if the lump was cancerous, allowed her to pause and recalibrate her options, and to take one step at a time. Giving herself permission to move slowly felt to her like the right decision. Talking about her experience months later, she had no regrets.

WHY REGRETS?

If there are no wrong decisions, can there be regrets? This question found its way into a study that I conducted many years ago but never got around to publishing. When participants showed up to the lab for the study, we told them we were running late and asked them to wait in an anteroom and come to the experimental room only when they saw a light on the wall flash green. We varied how we suggested they spend their time while they waited. One group was told we had *Seinfeld* episodes for them to watch, a second group was told to think about their feelings, a third group was given intentionally boring videos to watch, and the last group was asked to just wait. After twenty minutes, an experimenter returned to the anteroom and explained that other participants had come to the experimental room and had won a lot of money. "Joe made $150, Susan won $175." The experimenter then asked why those waiting hadn't come to the room. "The light never flashed green!" each of them excitedly explained. Then we asked how they felt about missing the opportunity to win money. It turned out that as long as an individual had spent the time well—enjoying *Seinfeld* or mindfully engaged in thought—they were pretty sanguine about the lost opportunity; they expressed no regret. But what about the others? They were angry and suffered regret. But they might not have made any money in the experiment, and they might have suffered embarrassment or other negative consequences.

Regret about a decision rests on a faulty assumption that the choice *not* made would have yielded more positive consequences. "This job is awful, I should have gone to the other firm," "The food here is tasteless, I should have gone to the other restaurant." But for all we know, the other firm or restaurant could have been even worse. And curiously, those who regret a decision are often the very people who believe the situation could always get worse. If it could have gotten worse, what sense does it make to regret one's choice? Our experience with the option not chosen will always be unknowable. We make a decision to take action. Once we take that action, we're different and can't assess what the alternative actions we could have taken would have felt like.

The way I see it, after a decision, whatever happens can have advantages. I look back on the fire described in chapter 2 and remember people's kindness. Even deciding to get into the Jeep in the Virgin Islands gave me something to talk and write about for years and helped me develop my decision-making theory.

NO RIGHT DECISIONS

The mindless belief that there is a single right decision not only creates stress but can take its toll on self-esteem. We beat ourselves up over our incompetence with questions like "Why am I so stupid? Why can't I make better decisions?" The result is that too many of us give control over our lives to others, so-called or self-appointed experts who seem to know how to make decisions better than we do. This may be dangerous if the expert hasn't got our best interest in mind. My view of decision-making relies on owning our actions, not relying on others to come up with the "right decision" for us.

The more we believe there is a right decision to be made, the harder it becomes to make decisions. Feedback is often scarce, and comparative feedback is often unavailable. Even if this were not the case, feedback still has to be interpreted, and a different interpretation could lead to a different decision. Should you marry? Last year / last month / yesterday, the person seemed perfect for you. Which side of the person's behavior is appealing or irritating? Is he trusting or gullible? If I see him as trusting, that's a plus. If I see him as gullible, that's a minus.

Whenever we can't decide, it's because the alternatives for us are not very different. If they appear the same, it doesn't matter what we choose. If the options seem different, meaning we have a preference, we should simply select it, with no calculation needed. But let's say you still want to go through a process of deciding. Assume you feel you have to choose between A and B. So, you start gathering information about the alternatives to make them look different. If you find out that A is a free trip to Paris and B is a free trip to the center of your town, you'd probably have a clear preference, and there would be no decision to make.

Decision-making in my view is really just information gathering until we arrive at a preference. Most people think when they gather information it'll tell them what to choose. But if we continue to search, each new piece of information could change that preference. Suppose there had just been a terrorist attack in Paris, you might choose not to go. Then you find out the trip could be taken any month or year over the next decade. And so on. After going back and forth with new information, we often become stressed and feel we should know what to choose already! But we really can't know. Decisions are always made in uncertainty and no matter how hard we try we cannot remove the uncertainty.

This is true even when it comes to serious medical decisions, such as our preferences regarding end-of-life care. We make decisions about the care we want if we become seriously ill before that happens, and essentially in the dark. We think we'll know what we want, but once we actually have to make choices, it's not unusual for people to change their minds and decide to continue living even if painful.

I agree with Dr. Damasio that our emotions color our perceptions and the information we choose to consider. But I think it's important to add that emotions also often determine what we deem as relevant in the first place. That is to say, just as in my decision as to where to start my academic career, the information gathered often follows the decision already made. I wanted to be in New York, and so I gathered information to make that the best choice for me.

GUESSES, PREDICTIONS, CHOICES, AND DECISIONS

If decisions don't require elaborate reasoning or even information gathering, what is the difference between *a guess, a prediction, a choice, and a decision*? We all know that when we're guessing it is because we don't know what the outcome will be. Similarly, when we make predictions, it's because we're unaware of what might be. Making a choice is no different. If there was no doubt, there would be no choice. Decisions are the same as each of these. In each case there are alternatives to be considered without a predetermined number of consequences to consider. In all cases, each consequence can be reasonably construed as positive or negative. When there is a decision to make, there is uncertainty. Without uncertainty, there is no need to decide. If you toss a biased coin that you know always comes up heads, you choose heads. If you're sure the operation will be successful, you have it without any further information gathering.

In my view the differences among guesses, predictions, choices, and decisions are the degrees of importance we assign to the outcomes rather than a difference in the process. How odd it would sound to say, "I guess I'll have the operation" or "I decided based on a coin toss." Yet, since we can't be sure the operation will be a success no matter how much information we gather, nor can we know all the potential consequences of having or not having it, our belief in the surgery to be a success is really no more than a guess. Knowing this may make health decisions a bit easier to make. Because the consequences can be life altering, however, we gather information to help us deal with the outcomes.

If the outcome is unimportant, we need not justify our decisions after the fact, but choosing what is important and what is trivial is very personal. Making decisions mindlessly can increase stress, and indecision or regret can reduce perceived control and lead to bad health outcomes. As previously discussed, the illusion of control is not an illusion from the actor's perspective. This would mean, ironically, then, that mindful decision-making even in chance situations may be good for our health.

I have argued that deciding and guessing are both made in equivalent uncertainty. Am I saying that deciding on medical treatments is the same as guessing about having a treatment? In a word, no. If we are deciding on a medical treatment, we will be noticing new things about the options, and that mindful noticing itself is good for our health. Thus, taking the time to decide between two health options should be better for our health than just guessing to have one versus the other. But mistakenly accepting the idea that decision-making is an objective pursuit, even in a medical context, is surely not the only nor indeed best way of becoming involved in our healthcare.

Let's go back to the illusion-of-control studies. We know that in general we spend more time with our decisions than with our guesses. We learn more about the alternatives and we take more control over our decisions than our guesses. Indeed, in the illusion-of-control studies, we found that the value of the lottery ticket depends on the owner having been encouraged to think about the ticket on multiple occasions. The bottom line is that the more effort and thought we put into something, the more control we feel we have.

The more we notice about something, the more we feel in control, and we notice more when we are deciding than when we are guessing. From a behavioral economics point of view, this seems irrational. The treatment I decided to have and the treatment I randomly chose may objectively be the same treatment, but psychologically they are quite different. Similarly, it seems irrational that we recover faster the more we pay for a pill, given it is the same pill in both instances, but research shows that we do indeed recover faster.

Sometimes our decisions appear irrational to other people, such as when our values and so our choices differ from theirs, when our preferences shift, when options appear different, and when options are contextualized differently as with the introduction of an irrelevant alternative, but all of this evaluating depends on a presumption of a correct decision. To that I say, "Who says so?" Once we realize the subjectivity of all of our decisions and give up the idea of objective probabilities and right and wrong, emotions like stress, regret, and negative feelings about our decision-making skill become less of a problem.

CHAPTER 5

Level Up

Healing is a matter of time, but it is sometimes
also a matter of opportunity.
—Hippocrates

Many of us make social comparisons on a daily basis, looking for how we are better or worse than someone else. *I'm thinner than she is now; she looks so much younger than I do. You got great tickets to a Broadway show when I had to stay home. I can't believe how much more money you have than I do. I'm a far better cook than he is.* More than once, I've seen a compliment given to one person make the person with them feel insulted by default. In making these social comparisons, over time we make ourselves miserable and unwilling to take up new activities for fear of coming up short. Interestingly, the negative effects of frequent social comparisons result whether we make downward (we are better) or upward (they are better) comparisons. Those who see themselves as better will at some point see themselves as worse. Research that my lab members Judith White, Leeat Yariv, Johnny Welch, and I conducted found that frequent social comparing was related to several destructive emotions and behaviors.[1] People who made frequent social comparisons were more likely to experience envy, guilt, regret, and defensiveness, and to lie, blame others, and have unmet cravings. Most important, I think, is that making social comparisons often leads to stress and sometimes depression. Thus, it has a negative impact on our health.

A famous social psychologist, Leon Festinger, believed we have a drive to make these comparisons, suggesting there is no other way to be.[2] I strongly disagree. There are many activities for which people don't make evaluative social comparisons. For example, most of us probably have never wondered if we are better or worse than someone else at brushing our teeth. Regardless, there is a compelling reason to avoid engaging in evaluative social comparing. Typically—and unwittingly—when we do so we are mindless, assuming there is a single understanding for why people behave as they do. Did they intend to do well or not really care? Was their behavior typical for them or was what you saw just an outlier? And was the criteria for the evaluation the only way to judge their performance?

Understandably, when we encounter a new phenomenon, an unexpected behavior, or try to understand other people, we look to come up with explanations and interpretations for it. When mindless, we tend to jump to the first conclusion; when mindful, we are able to imagine multiple explanations and perspectives and keep them in mind as possibilities without deciding which one is best.

When I was a graduate student, I attended a lecture by Yale

social psychology professor Bill McGuire. He was perhaps best known for his work on persuasion, but he was also astute when it came to understanding how psychologists can be wrong in interpreting behavior.[3] Sometimes, he pointed out, people engage in the very same behavior but for different reasons. Sometimes they look the same but are really quite different. This was his example: There are people who don't read *The New Yorker,* people who read *The New Yorker,* and people who don't read it any longer. People in the first and the third group look the same—none of them are reading the magazine—but they are very different people, and our research should distinguish between them. We could include another group of people, of course, who have started to read it again, and the same point would be made. Now the second and the fourth group misleadingly look the same.

To me, this way of thinking went far beyond just those studying behavior. I think it is common for virtually all of us. I went on to think of the many examples of what I came to think of as Level 1-2-3 thinking. A woman drops her walking cane as she passes by three people. Person A doesn't help her because he is just not a nice person. Person B tries to help her because she values kindness and assistance. Person C doesn't help her because he believes the woman will ultimately feel better if she picks it up herself and becomes more self-reliant. From the perspective of person B, both person A and person C appear to be heartless, uncaring bystanders. But in fact, they have almost entirely opposite motivations.

Most of the time, when people look to explain something, they mindlessly find a single explanation and stop their search. We've successfully run studies on adults and children to increase their mindfulness by having them come up with several explanations for a single event or behavior.

For example, you see a man taking money out of a cash register. Why might he be doing that? He could be a thief. He could be the cashier, making change. He could be the owner, withdrawing the day's earnings. He could be a repairman fixing the cash register. He could be an auditor, doing a spot inspection.

The point is we don't know. Being mindful about our interpretation—noticing new things—helps us become aware of the inherent uncertainty in our experience of the world. One might program a computer to continuously notice new things—say, a motion detector—but obviously that wouldn't make the computer mindful. When a person is mindful, she begins to realize there are things she doesn't know or knew incorrectly.

Level 1-2-3 thinking offers us a way to change the mindsets that limit us by applying multiple perspectives. It ranks how mindful our explanations are. Level 1 is the state in which we see things naïvely and know we don't know. Level 2 describes the state in which we think we are acting rationally, and typically become certain of our understandings, and level 3 is the state in which we are being mindful, applying multiple perspectives. Once we see that anything can be explained in many ways, we recognize and accept the inherent uncertainty. Being aware that these levels of thought exist is the first step toward helping us discover new, mindful explanations of our behavior and that of others. For any possible explanation, it brings us to ask, what other interpretations might exist?

I'm not suggesting that Level 1-2-3 is a step-by-step strategy. It's not as though you start at 1, then go to 2, and then progress to 3, and you're mindful. Instead, it is more a measure or description of how people inherently approach a particular situation. Level 2 thinking is essentially mindless. At this level, people think they know. Everything is always changing, and everything looks different from different perspectives, so this absolute knowing is a fiction. As a result, they are frequently in error while rarely in doubt. Once we accept that there may be several equally good explanations for any behavior, however, we may be able to move past level 2 to level 3 thinking and become more mindful. It is not just that our relationships improve now that we've gained a more nuanced explanation of the meaning of other people's behavior; we know from more than forty years of research that mindfulness is literally and figuratively enlivening. That is, since level 3 thinking is mindful, it is good for our health.

One of my pet peeves is the way people at level 2 respond to new inventions, or progress of any sort. With level 2 thinking, people can come to believe that progress comes in bursts: As soon as there is a breakthrough, many presume that's as good as it can get, at least for a while. My view is somewhat different. More improvement is always available.

Consider Zeno's paradox regarding distance.[4] Zeno posited that if you always move half the distance from where you are to where you want to be, you'll never get there. If you're only a foot away, then you'll be half a foot away, then a quarter of a foot away, and so on into smaller and smaller distances—but always a distance away, however tiny.

A level 1 view of Zeno's paradox would be to ignore the logic and just rely on our horse sense: Obviously we always get to where we want to go.

A level 2 view would accept the logical argument and try to solve it.

A level 3 view might accept the truth of the logical argument but see it in a different light, namely, that there is always a step toward our goal that we can reach if we continue to break it down by halves. Consider dieting. If you think you can't stop eating the whole box of cookies, remember Zeno, and leave half the box. If you can't leave half, leave a quarter, and so on. Everyone can, at the very least, eat one crumb fewer, which gives us a new starting point to begin the exercise again. Each time we see that we can do what we originally thought we couldn't do, we get a new perspective regarding what is possible.

Or consider free will. Suppose I'm choosing whether to take the A train or the D train to get home. After some light exercise of free will and some thoughtful contemplation, I actively choose D, and make it home safe and sound. Later, I learn that the A train was shut down the whole time anyway, so I would have had to take the D train no matter what. Did I have free will in the choice of the D train?

Both the level 1 and level 3 thinkers would say yes, while level 2 would say no. But the level 1 and level 3 thinkers would be saying yes for different reasons. The level 1 approach might lead one to say, "Well, I thought about it, and I made a choice. Who cares if the alternative turned out not to be available? The choice is what matters." Or even more likely, the level 1 thinker might simply declare that they do indeed have free will. Level 2 thinkers would say that free will in this case was an illusion because it could not have changed the train I ended up on. Level 3 thinkers might expand the choices available beyond just taking the A or D train and say, how else might I have gotten home? The choices are far wider than just the A or the D train. I could have walked. I could have taken a taxi or a bus. I could have rented a car. I could have chosen to go somewhere else entirely, or to spend the night in the subway station. Or I could have taken the D train reluctantly.

As we've seen, events don't have values assigned to them. Things are only what we make of them. Using level 3 thinking means I'm empowered by knowing that I have many alternatives available to me. Hence free will is no illusion.

All of us can employ the range of Level 1-2-3 thinking in our everyday experiences. We see a preteen acting without inhibition, say, singing loudly in the supermarket, and perhaps we assume they haven't yet learned the prevailing social norms. When we see an adult behaving just like the adolescent, we need to ask whether he is childishly uninhibited or whether he knows the rules and chooses to disregard them. Rather than being childishly uninhibited, perhaps he is maturely disinhibited.

Not infrequently, elderly adults may be misunderstood in this way. Children might want ice cream all the time; adults know that it's not supposed to be good for us to eat too much sugar. Surely a ninety-five-year-old should be able to decide for herself. Perhaps painkillers should be limited because of the possibility of becoming addicted. Should we limit the amount of morphine taken by a ninety-eight-year-old who is in pain?

Moreover, we should be careful when we evaluate someone

behaving in a "bad" way, as there are probably multiple explanations for why it is actually a "good" way, at least in some contexts (and at least to them). Additionally, if you are doing something for one reason and I'm doing it for another, what sense does a social comparison make in the first place? I'm passing up the pizza because I'm allergic to tomatoes, and you're not eating it because you're trying to diet. Is one of us better than the other?

TRYING OR DOING?

The realization that the same behavior can be understood in a way that may seem feeble (level 1) or lofty (level 3) is important both personally and interpersonally when viewed from a normative level 2.

Let's say that three students are writing a paper. The first one is not trying, just going through the motions. The second is trying, and you can see the enormous effort he or she is expending. The third person is, like the first person, not sweating at all, because he or she is simply doing, not "trying."

At first glance, the first and third both look carefree, but for entirely different reasons. Doing something effortlessly can often look like you're doing something without sufficient exertion or care. In both cases, onlookers may complain that you're not even trying because the behavior looks the same, even if it has different motivations.

To be sure, it is better to try than to give up or just go through the motions. But even better would be to *just do*. You wouldn't tell a child to try to eat his ice cream.

When you are told to try, or you tell yourself to try, you implicitly acknowledge that failure is a real possibility. When you "just do it," you focus on process rather than outcome. Yoda was correct when he said, "Do or do not. There is no try."

Lab member Kris Nichols and I are now doing research on how students respond to a request to try to do something, versus to simply do something.[5] If you tell students to try to do some difficult problems, they tend to perform worse than if you simply tell them to do what is required. For example, in one study with Harvard undergraduates we investigated the effects of framing a task as something participants should either try or do. We hypothesized that when people frame their efforts around the word "try," they are preparing themselves for the possibility that they might fail and that they will perform worse on tasks because of this. We predicted that when people frame their tasks with "doing" as the active verb, they are more singularly focused on the task at hand and will perform better.

In the study, ninety-two participants answered seven questions from the LSAT law admission test that measure logical and verbal reasoning. Shortly before the test, participants were instructed to either "do" or "try" the test. Data confirmed our primary hypothesis—participants who were told to "Do the LSAT" answered significantly more questions correctly (an average of 4.52 tasks of the 7 we gave them) than participants who were told to "Try to Do the LSAT" (an average of 3).

Maybe you're wondering about the idea of *hoping* to do something. It turns out that hope is not unlike *trying*. At first pass it looks positive. It is surely better to be hopeful rather than hopeless, but to use the Level 1-2-3 analogy, there is a third, better-than-better way: Do. Hope carries with it both the seed of doubt and also the stress endemic to it. When we wake up and walk to the kitchen for caffeine, for instance, we don't "hope" to get a cup of coffee. To do so would plant the seed of doubt about its availability. No, we head to the kitchen for our coffee and our action—the doing of it—assumes it'll be there.

BLAME AND FORGIVENESS

If you've ever accidentally stepped on your dog's foot, you might have been surprised with how quickly the animal will try to make you feel better. There's no hesitation, no blame, no anger, just immediate reconciliation. The range of reactions from a human on whose foot you've stepped doesn't often include reconciliation. Anger, annoyance, or even a shove, yes. Maybe even a grudge held for decades.

Dogs are onto something. Forgiveness is better than holding a grudge. It's a more elevated way of thinking about the situation. But there is still a better way. Bear in mind that one cannot forgive without first blaming. And even though forgiveness is almost universally regarded as a good thing by virtually all societies and religions, blame is equally universally regarded as a bad thing. Yet one cannot exist without the other. Every forgiver must also be a blamer.

It gets worse. What do we blame people for, good outcomes or bad outcomes? We tend to blame only for bad outcomes. But outcomes do not come with sticky notes from the heavens specifying whether they are good or bad. It is up to us to classify and take views of events. So, who ultimately forgives? People who first view the world negatively, then blame, and then forgive? Hardly divine.

Forgiveness is better than blame, but there is a better-than-better, level 3, way: understanding. When you understand someone's behavior from their perspective, there is no need to blame, and there is nothing to forgive.

You invite a couple for dinner at seven o'clock, but they don't show up until eight o'clock. One option we have is to view their lateness as a disrespectful affront to the value of our time and dinner preparation, and we spend the hour stewing and blaming. Then, when they arrive, we give them a haughty look and wait. We wait for their prostration and judge the sincerity of their apologies. After a pause, we magnanimously forgive. Was our evening well spent?

We have another option. Assuming we can dispel mindless worry about their whereabouts or anxiety about overcooking their meal when they don't arrive at seven o'clock, we can look at it as though they have given us a gift. We can return some phone calls we've been putting off or make some progress on a show or series we've been watching. We can paint or surf the Web or read a book or take a nap. When they do arrive, we can thank them. How often do we find a stolen hour of free time? There is no negativity, no blame, and nothing to forgive.

When you take the better-than-better path of understanding, you start to appreciate that every negative aspect of a person's behavior is also a positive. As discussed in chapter 3, someone who is always late may be considered unreliable, but they may also be seen as flexible. Someone who is gullible is also trusting; someone who is grim is also serious. In fact, every negative ascription has an equally potent but oppositely valanced alternative.

When you understand someone mindfully, there is no need for blame. You can appreciate and be happy for your friends' spontaneity and look forward to hearing what latest adventures deterred them for an hour today. In fact, whenever we are being judgmental, we are blind to a better way. Once we realize that an action makes sense from the actor's perspective or else she wouldn't have done it, negative judgments tend to disappear. Rather than dislike me because I am gullible, perhaps you'll appreciate me for being so trusting. From the actor's perspective, inconsistent is flexible, impulsive is spontaneous, grim is serious, distracted is otherwise attracted, and lazy is insufficiently motivated.

I'm reminded of an experience my sister's friend had many years ago when she was teaching elementary school. There were two brothers in her class who never attended on the same day. At first, she wondered whether they were being disrespectful, which was a kind of level 1 interpretation of their absence. Then she decided to just accept the disrespect, level 2. Eventually, she found out that they had only one pair of shoes to share—and understood there was no need for her negative judgment.

Mindful reasoning may also be applied to loneliness. One of the silver linings of lockdowns and quarantines may have been that many people independently discovered the level 3 way of thinking about social isolation. Pre-Covid, a level 1 person was alone but lonely. A level 2 person was socializing and mingling with people. But a level 3 person was alone and content. Many activities such as writing, painting, or playing single-player video games are better alone. We may think we need a cure for loneliness, but what we really need are ways to actively engage ourselves.

Level 1-2-3 thinking is pertinent to how we integrate work and "life" too. Discussions of the importance of work-life balance imply that we, by necessity, are different people depending on whether we are at work being stressed or at home relaxing with our families.

I believe we should seek work/life integration rather than work/life balance. At level 1, people work and ignore the rest of living, often assuming they'll get to enjoy themselves eventually. At level 2, people realize the importance of life outside of work and struggle to balance both. At level 3 people integrate work and life, realizing that much of what "life" provides can be gotten at work. This is true even for what many consider menial work.

I went to visit a friend who lived in the very posh Museum Tower in New York City. Although there is no longer a need for an elevator operator, this building had one. I thought how boring it must be for him. Then he challenged my assumption. He made it a bit of a game for himself in guessing how long it would take the elevator to get to our destination, which happened to be the thirty-third floor. Rather than turn his wheel and watch the numbers light up as the elevator ascended, he looked away and guessed how long it would take to get to my destination. He looked back at the display at the thirtieth floor.

With a level 3 approach, we become less judgmental. At level 1 you don't know enough to judge, at level 2 you judge, and then at level 3 you don't judge anymore. Evaluative social comparisons no longer make any sense. As we become less judgmental, our relationships improve, and as research by social psychologists has made clear, social support is good for our health.

We typically can't know if a person is at level 1 or level 3 since they look alike. When your dog "reconciles" with you after you step on his paw, is he being naïve and unable to understand the concept of blame and forgiveness? Of course, we don't know what if anything the dog is thinking. But if we assume it's a level 3 response such that he assumes it was an accident so there's nothing to forgive, we can learn from him and we can grow regardless of whether the "forgiveness" was a level 1 or a level 3.

Thus, if someone was at a level 1 but we viewed them as a level 3, we might first accept a better way of understanding behavior by recognizing a more elevated alternative. Second, we might improve our relationship with this person. And third, we would be likely to treat them more kindly, which could, in turn, elevate their behavior. Moreover, when we stop mindlessly judging others, we become less likely to continue judging ourselves.

FINDING MEANING

One of the most important applications of this Level 1-2-3 way of thinking may be to finding meaning in our lives. In a level 1 way of thinking, meaning is considered extrinsic. We make choices, but they are relatively minor ones. If we want a child to eat eggs, for example, we don't ask them an open-ended question about what they want. We ask them if they want their eggs scrambled or boiled. They have a choice, but it is limited.

Much of my early life was spent in this way of thinking. I made relatively minor decisions like what to major in and which schools to apply to, but my "track" felt set. Get great grades. Please my teachers and then professors. Continue on that path.

Why did I go into psychology in the first place? I was a straight-A student so at least by conventional measures I was good at most things academic. But I really enjoyed Professor Philip Zimbardo's introduction to psychology course and thought, why not, I'll major in psychology. Did I pursue a long, mindful introspection on what meaning my life would have had if I had pursued chemistry, my original major, instead? Not really. Even choosing which schools to apply to, both as a student and as a professor, were relatively safe choices. Which ones are the best? Okay, I'll apply there. I was answering scrambled or boiled, but who was asking how I like my eggs? It was something extrinsic.

A level 2 way of thinking about the course of my life might have led me to rigidly evaluate the net present value of my wealth across different conditions depending on my choices of majors, fields of study, and even occupation. But as we have seen, level 2 thinking is also typically mindless.

Indeed, level 2 thinking has a drawback that level 1 does not: disappointment. The level 1 way of thinking about the meaning of life is to not really think about it at all. We can live micro-mindfully, and do the tasks assigned to us in a mindful way, and that's certainly better than doing them in a mindless way. But we could also mindfully consider our situation. From the level 2 approach, we think we'll be happy once we start dating, or once we get a car, or once we're married, or once we're divorced, or once we move to New York, or once we get that job, or once we leave that job, or once we retire. It's a road too often filled with disappointment, because each completed task is a letdown. With enough such letdowns, we may begin to feel as if life has no meaning whatsoever.

Can a level 3 approach lead us out of this morass? Let's remember Zeno and the lesson that because everything is potentially meaningless (or unreachable, in Zeno's paradox), everything is also potentially meaningful.

We have to choose to impose meaning ourselves. It is not extrinsic. A level 3 way of thinking would recognize that we can make changes at any point because nothing has inherent meaning. Should we retire at sixty-five? Ninety? Never? These are all possibilities. Should you be an astronaut or a piano player? A baseball player or a physicist? Or all of the above? Why not?

I think, right now, that I could be happy as a novelist. I've never written a novel. But why not? Mindfully engaging in the writing process comes with its own rewards, even if I never finish it.

The existential realization that there may not be any external meaning or purpose to anything can be devastating, but it can also be liberating. It can free us all up to enjoy whatever we are doing.

CHAPTER 6

Mind and Body as One

So the problem is not so much to see what nobody has
yet seen, as to think what nobody has yet thought
concerning that which everybody sees.
—ARTHUR SCHOPENHAUER

A view of the body as distinct from the mind, inexorably running its course through illness and aging, puts unnecessary limits on our lives. Understanding the unity of mind and body can, like questioning rules and risks, or realizing that resources may not be limited, give us greater control, and open up avenues once seen as impossible.

The first time I recognized the unity of mind and body I was in a restaurant on my honeymoon in Paris. I ordered a mixed grill. Everything on the plate was sure to be delicious except the *ris de veau* (sweetbread, or pancreas), but I was determined to eat it regardless. I was nineteen going on thirty and trying to be ever so sophisticated—after all, I was now a married woman. The plate arrived, and I asked my new husband which of the grilled items was the pancreas. I ate everything else on the plate. Now the dreaded moment came. I tried to eat it but was getting more and more nauseated. Meanwhile, a very big smile spread over his face. I asked him what was so funny about my feeling sick. I then learned that I'd eaten the pancreas a while ago and what I was having such difficulty eating was chicken.

At that moment a theory was born, although it would take years for me to articulate it.

MIND-BODY DUALISM

Anyone who has grown nauseated at the sight of someone vomiting has had firsthand experience of the mind influencing the body. Still, our entire Western tradition of thought sees them as separate.

Although Aristotle believed that a quiet and happy mind makes the body healthy, Plato and other classical Greek philosophers viewed the mind and body as fundamentally distinct entities with limited interaction. Descartes's view of mind-body dualism became the accepted model for medicine in the West. When Robert Koch, a bacteriologist, found the cause of anthrax, along with identifying the bacteria that caused tuberculosis and cholera, our dualistic view was strengthened. Around that same time, Louis Pasteur developed vaccinations for rabies and anthrax and showed that disease is caused by "germs," and not bad air as was previously believed. Clearly these were discoveries of great importance.

Unfortunately, they also led to the presumption of one-way causation for disease. In that model, illness relies on the introduction of a pathogen, which then causes physical systems to go awry. Psychological variables may play a minor role in health but matters of mind and matters of body unfold in parallel, neither affecting the other. Disease in this model is seen as a purely physiological process, and treatment operates on the disease state at that level. Thoughts and emotions do not cause disease.

Early ideas regarding health in the East, however, were more holistic. As early as A.D. 600, Indian texts talked of a strong relationship between mental state and disease—hate, violence, and grief were all thought to upset health. Traditional Chinese medicine, which has been around for more than two thousand years, also recognized the effect our minds can have on our bodies. Indeed, this tradition emphasizes the importance of chi (life force) and seeks to stoke it to achieve optimal health. Evolving from these early Asian ideas, holistic medicine today emphasizes treating the body with nutrition, exercise, herbal remedies, aromatherapy, and other complementary therapies.

Although some still accept the medical model, the biosocial model of illness is now the prevalent view. Developed by George Engel, it recognizes that biological (genetic, biochemical), psychological (personality, emotion, cognition), and social factors (family, culture) interact to cause illness, and hence the mind can affect the body.[1] Still, a fundamental belief in mind-body dualism—that mind and body are separate, even if they affect one another—continues. Researchers continue to devote their efforts to finding meditating links between psychological and physical experiences. This is driven home to me every time I submit a research paper and the reviewers ask what accounts for the health results. They are asking, "How can you get from this fuzzy thing called a thought to something material called a body?" The underlying assumption, of course, is that mind and body are separate, and thus the cause cannot be "just" psychological.

A MORE COMPLETE MIND-BODY UNITY

As you will recall from the introduction to this book, some of my early research helped set the stage for what came to be called mind-body medicine. My nursing home study showed that when elderly adults were encouraged to make decisions or care for a plant, they were twice as likely as controls to be alive eighteen months later.[2] About the same time, psychologists Richard Schulz and Barbara Hanusa found that giving nursing home elders control over when they would receive visitors affected longevity.[3] Nursing home studies in which we offered memory training likewise increased longevity.[4] These longevity effects were also found in a study comparing our mindful "active noticing" treatment to Transcendental Meditation. (While my early research concerned meditation, almost all of my work now looks at mindfulness without meditation.)[5]

Armed with data showing that psychological interventions may affect longevity, we started testing the concept of mind-body unity. Think of your arm. You can see and experience it as an arm or as a wrist, elbow, upper arm, or forearm. But by moving any part of your arm, you move or affect all of the parts that make up your arm. Even when you think you are just moving your wrist, your entire arm is affected—in fact, your entire body is affected. It is not that the wrist affects the arm. The wrist is part of the arm. In the same way, *every thought affects every part of the body.* We may not have the technology now to see all the effects, but one day we may. We now know, for example, that a teardrop of joy is biochemically different from a teardrop from cutting an onion. And there are data showing that growth marks in our baby teeth may reveal mental health and depression when we get older. That is, childhood stress and adversity affect dental enamel.

Research by the Israeli scientist Asya Rolls shows that our immune responses begin in the brain.[6] When she induced abdominal inflammation in mice, she found that certain neurons in the brain were activated. Scientists later were able to produce the same inflammation by stimulating these neurons. As Dr. Rolls has said, "Somehow there are these 'thoughts' that initiate real physiological processes."[7]

Her research also showed that positive expectations can boost antibacterial and anti-tumor immunity: When pleasure centers in the brain were stimulated, tumor growth slowed.[8] The point is that immune responses are shaped by the brain. Inhibit the relevant neurons and disease symptoms lessen.

Any change is virtually simultaneously occurring in every cell of our bodies. If I lift my arm, there are differences in my brain from before I lifted it. If I have a thought about my dog, my brain has changed from before the thought. Rather than assume that while our minds are engaged, our physiology is inactive, or vice versa, seeing it as one implies that thought and bodily responses occur simultaneously. One might ask, "If I lose a limb or weight, does that mean I lose part of my mind?" The argument is mind-body unity, not mind-body equality;

your mind is certainly affected by your lost limb or change in weight, it's just not one-for-one. One might also ask, "If my mind keeps changing, does that mean my body does so as well?" The simple answer is yes. The body regenerates all the time.

The psychology department at Harvard has what we call Harvest Day, when many of the faculty give a brief lecture about their current work. After I spoke about my research on mind-body unity, one of my respected colleagues asked, "What's going on under the hood?" referring to the *neuroscience* of mind-body unity. What's happening at the level of the brain, he wanted to know. What is the chain of events from a thought to changes in the body? Of course, this question has plagued philosophers for centuries.

For me, mind-body unity means that neurological changes are happening more or less simultaneously rather than sequentially. Moreover, the changes are happening throughout our bodies—even if scientists choose only to look at the brain. We can make bodily changes by changing our minds without regard to what's happening under the hood. We needn't wait to change our bodies; we can do that right now.

TESTING MIND-BODY UNITY

My first test of this radical concept was conducted in 1979, in my counterclockwise study.[9] To recap: Our aim was to see if priming the minds of elderly men to believe that they were in the past would also affect their bodies. To do that we had the men leave their homes to live in a retreat for a week. The retreat had been retrofitted to resemble life twenty years earlier—in every way possible. They watched news broadcasts and other television shows and movies of that era, listened to jukebox favorites, and were asked to talk about it all in the present tense, as if these things were happening in real time. A control group lived at the same retreat for a week discussing the same topics, but in the past tense.

Before the retreat, we measured a number of biological, psychological, and physical markers in the men. We found that after spending time in a novel, stimulating environment, the scores for biological, psychological, and physical status improved over baseline on several measures for both groups. Likewise, hearing, memory, and grip strength improved. Nevertheless, the experimental group outperformed the control group on many other measures. Vision, joint flexibility, manual dexterity, IQ, gait, and posture improved, and symptoms of arthritis decreased. These findings were remarkable, since hearing or vision, for example, rarely improve without medical intervention in any age group and especially in an older population. More recently, my postdocs Francesco Pagnini, Deborah Phillips, and I replicated the counterclockwise study in Italy by having people live as if they were their younger selves, acting as if they were living in the year 1989.[10] Again, we found improved physical function.

In further research testing mind-body unity, we looked at other kinds of cues that can prime health-related effects. Take age-related cues around clothing. Advertisements show us who certain styles are "made for" and store design perpetuates the notion of what's "age appropriate"; miniskirts aren't sold in many stores meant for women my age, and if I were at a store trying them on, I'm sure I'd get disparaging looks from the saleswomen. Far from simply being annoying and ageist, these cues can have effects on our health. Consider uniforms, which tend to remove age-related cues; when people are wearing uniforms at work, they are not subtly reminded of their age. In one study I did with then students Jaewoo Chung and Laura Hsu, we controlled for things like status and pay and found that those who regularly wear uniforms live longer.[11] While I can't assume that age-related cues and the negative expectations those cues elicit were the sole reason for the extended lives of our subjects, I think it's reasonable to make the link.

But it turns out that we don't need external physical cues to benefit from a change in how young we think we look and the corresponding change that may be seen on measures of health. In another study, we photographed women and measured their blood pressure before and after they got a haircut. In both sets of photos, however, we covered their hair so all they could see were their faces.

Then we asked the women to evaluate their appearance in each photo. We asked them if they thought they looked younger in the later photos. For many of the women, the mere fact of having had a haircut (they knew which photo was "before" and which was "after") convinced them that they did indeed look younger. What's more, people who we brought in to judge the photos independently agreed that they looked younger afterward. And for these women there was a health benefit to believing that they looked younger, since their blood pressure had also decreased.

To test the effects of perception on physiology, I conducted an experiment with hotel chambermaids with Alia Crum when she was my student at Harvard (she is now a professor at Stanford).[12] While the work of chambermaids is physically strenuous, our participants did not see it as exercise because "exercise" was seen to happen before or after work. We wanted to know whether the work might have a different effect on their bodies if they conceived of it as exercise. Participants were randomly divided into two groups, one given only general health information. The experimental group was taught that their work was exercise, comparing it to work on specific machines and exercises one finds in a gym. (Making a bed was like working on a rowing machine, while mopping provided a good upper body workout.) There were no discernible differences with respect to how hard or long the chambermaids worked nor what or how much they ate over the monthlong intervention. The only difference was whether they now believed their work was exercise. As a result of this change in mindset, the experimental group showed significant changes: They lost weight, their body mass index declined, their blood pressure came down, and their waist-to-hip ratio decreased.

When I lecture about our chambermaid study, I show a slide of two women at the gym just to make sure the audience understands what I'm saying. One is on a stationary bicycle and the other is standing nearby talking to her. I tell them that if the exercising woman sees herself just as socializing rather than exercising, she probably won't benefit much from the exercise. If the non-exercising woman, however, sees herself as having spent the day at the gym, she could still experience some of the benefits of exercise.

Mind-body unity means that everything we do, experience,

or think is relevant to our health. If we go to a baseball game and are happy that our team won, if we try a new restaurant and fight with a waiter who appears to be ignoring us, or if we watch a funny television program, each of the activities are registered in our bodies, and they affect our health moment by moment, day in, day out. Small changes in living our life mindfully add up.

POWERS OF PERCEPTION

Alia Crum took this research one step further. She and a colleague at Stanford, Octavia Zahrt, surveyed more than sixty thousand people over twenty-one years old, controlling for things such as health and demographic factors.[13] The surveys included questions about how much exercise individuals thought they were getting relative to other people their own age. Crum and Zahrt found a significant relationship between the *perception* of activity and mortality. People who did not perceive themselves as active were more likely to die in the period of the study than those who believed they had been active. This was true regardless of the actual amount of exercise they got.

Other researchers have found similar results. Abiola Keller and her colleagues at Marquette University have shown that it is not stress that is harmful as much as the *perception* that stress is harmful.[14] Adults who perceived that stress was harmful and reported experiencing a good deal of stress were more likely to die earlier than those adults who did not report high levels of stress. What is surprising is that the longevity of those who to many people lived stressful lives but did not perceive that stress was harmful was no different from those whose lives were not significantly stressed.

When I was a first-year graduate student we were introduced to the labs of many of the psychology department's professors. In one lab the professor studied taste and shared with us the existence of a substance that had the effect of making things that had a good deal of sugar in them taste sour and another substance that made food that was sour taste sweet. It was strange indeed to eat something I expected would be sweet but instead recoil at its sourness. Ever since then, I have wondered whether if I consume something that artificially tastes sweet, would my body respond to the "idea" of sweetness or would it respond to what I actually consumed? Would my blood sugar level increase, even though I did not eat sugar? Mind-body unity theory would predict the idea would be more powerful than the actuality.

While it is yet to be done, one of the strongest tests of the influence of perception would be a study comparing the long-term health of heavy smokers who believe that smoking causes cancer, emphysema, or COPD with those who truly don't believe it or those who believe obesity is a killer compared with those who don't. If believing you'll become ill leads to illness, the reason could be either that the belief makes it so or that engaging in a behavior seen as dangerous is stressful and stress is the killer.

Of course, belief about the dangers of a habit is difficult to measure. But sleep—how much you get—is a measurable act. How malleable our perceptions are of our sleep patterns is also quantifiable. People from the medical school at Harvard joined members of my lab and me to conduct a study on sleep. Our intervention was simple: We programmed a bedside clock to alter the amount of time that participants thought they had slept, irrespective of their actual sleep duration.[15]

When the clock was sped up, such that people thought they had slept for eight hours but had slept only for five, their reaction times were quicker on an auditory psychomotor vigilance test as compared to their performance when knew they had five hours of sleep. Conversely, when people slept for eight hours but thought that they only slept for five, their performance was worse than when they had slept eight hours and thought they had slept eight hours. Clearly, our perceptions of how much we've slept, and not just the actual number of hours, matter.

These perceptions also influenced brain activity, a more objective measure of alertness and relaxation. Participants wore an EEG (electroencephalography) cap to record their brainwaves, which are oscillations in neural activity. When people are alert, their brain activity registers as a frequency known as alpha waves. In the study, these alpha waves correlated more with the participants' perceptions of how much they slept rather than their actual sleep duration. For example, when people thought their sleep was cut short, their brains appeared to be less alert. This was true for a variety of physical measurements. In other words, the perception of sleep being restricted makes our brain act as if sleep was restricted.

Mind-body unity suggests that fatigue itself may be under our control. I discussed fatigue in my book *Counterclockwise*, where I asserted that fatigue may be determined by our mind, not biological physical limits.[16] That is, mental and physical energy are not governed by different underlying processes, as many assume. They're not separate biological functions. If this is true, then we may have a good deal of control over whether or not we get tired. I described two informal studies we did back then. I asked people in one of my classes to ask their friends to do either 100 or 200 jumping jacks and ask them to tell them when they got tired. Both groups reported that they experienced fatigue about two-thirds of the way through the activity. That means that the first group got tired after about 65–70 jumping jacks, but the second group didn't get tired until after about 130–140. In another informal experiment, we had people type one or two pages without stopping using a word-processing program that gave them no feedback regarding errors. For the one-page group, the most errors occurred around two-thirds of the way through. Although the second group typed twice as much, their errors didn't appear until two-thirds of the way through the two pages. We impose a structure on the tasks we do so that we have a sense of a beginning, a middle, and an end.

When I used to drive from Boston to New Haven, I got antsy and tired as I approached Southbridge, Massachusetts—the halfway point. On the other hand, when I drove to New York City, twice the distance away, I was fine until I got close to Hartford, Connecticut—about halfway to New York and farther than Southbridge.

Members of my lab and I recently ran several studies to more formally test the idea that fatigue is a mental construct: The first one assessed fatigue in a long-distance travel study.

The second study looked at fatigue in a boring counting study. In the third and fourth studies we had people engage in physical tasks to assess the same hypothesis.[17]

It turns out that my driving experience was not unique. Based on self-reports, participants indicated that they, on average, started experiencing fatigue about 50 percent of the way through their travels and experienced the most fatigue around 75 percent of the way through their travel regardless of the actual amount of time they spent traveling in their car.

In the counting study, we wanted to see if brain waves follow this same pattern. When participants came to our laboratory, we seated them in front of a computer, placed the NeuroSky MindWave EEG headset on their head, and instructed them to follow the instructions on the computer screen. They were then randomly assigned to one of the three experimental groups: (a) 200-counting task, (b) 400-counting task, or (c) 600-counting task. In the 200-counting task, we gave participants a sheet with 200 randomly generated integers between 1 and 80. They were instructed to use a pencil to mark each number that was a multiple of 3. In the other two conditions, the instructions and procedures were the same, but now there were either 400 randomly generated integers between 1 and 80, or 600 randomly generated integers between 1 and 80. Participants in all three conditions were told that they had fifteen minutes to complete the task. Thus, we varied the mental load of the task without varying the length of the task. We know that people make mistakes when they are tired, so we used the number of mistakes made as our primary measure of fatigue. Most of the mistakes were at the halfway point in each group. That is, people in the first group made mistakes at around 100, but people in the second group didn't make mistakes until they reached 200. Finally, those in the 600 group didn't make mistakes until around 300. The EEG data show the same effect. Observable peaks of compensation signals in alpha band EEG wave amplitude were observed for the subjects during the fatigue periods.

In the next study we simply had people squeeze a hand grip for 120 seconds, 180 seconds, or 240 seconds and report when they got tired. Again, we found that fatigue depended on how long they expected to hold the grip, rather than on how long they actually held it.

The next study in the series also assessed physical fatigue and was conducted with ballerinas from the Hessisches Staatsballett in Wiesbaden, Germany. Ballerinas are a population accustomed to pursuing a task in the face of pain and physical and mental exhaustion. They work five to six days a week, with full workdays consisting of training in the morning and rehearsing through to the evening. Their bodies are trained to withstand physical discomfort, and their stamina aids in the completion of two-to-three-hour performances in the face of blisters, painful joints and muscles, and, in some cases, serious injuries.

Our study was of a dance move called a *développé à la seconde*, which involves holding the leg fully extended (that is, without a bent knee) off the ground to the side, typically at a ninety-degree angle or higher. From a pilot study with both female and male professional ballet dancers from the Atlanta Ballet, we already knew the average hold time of this move, so we knew approximately how long most of the German dancers might stay in the pose.

We made video recordings of the participants' *développé* tasks and asked three observers who were trained professional dancers (not informed about the study) to watch each video recording with a stopwatch and record in seconds when they believed the videoed dancer (a) *started* experiencing fatigue, and (b) when he or she experienced the *most* fatigue. Again, we found support for our hypothesis. The results indicated that neither the duration of the task nor the gender of the participant determined our observers' notation of when the participants started experiencing fatigue. The dancers began to show signs of experiencing fatigue about one-third of the way through the ballet position hold, and their fatigue peaked about three-quarters of the way through the ballet position.

When we do a task mindlessly, our expectations determine whether we'll be tired. It doesn't matter if we think we'll get tired one-third, halfway, or two-thirds of the way through it. The point is the same. Our fatigue often may be determined by our minds, not physical limits.

In another important study that supports mind-body unity and this view of fatigue, Alia Crum and her colleagues performed genetic testing to determine whether participants had a gene that predisposes them to getting tired easily.[18] Subjects ran on a treadmill until they were tired to get baseline scores. Then she randomly divided them into two groups. Half were told they had the "tiring" gene and half were told they did not have it. Thus, some were given accurate information—they had the gene or did not have it—and some were told they had it even though they did not. Everyone ran again on the treadmill one week later. The researchers found that beliefs controlled their performance, regardless of their genes. Those who believed they had poorer genes had less endurance and poorer lung capacity, and there was a change in metabolic exchange rate, which means they were less effective at ridding their bodies of carbon dioxide.

The idea of structuring the tasks we do with a clear beginning, middle, and end serves a purpose. It allows us to complete one thing so we can move on to a different task. Nevertheless, it appears that this structure is malleable. Knowing that we essentially control when we get tired can enable us to willfully change when doing so is to our advantage.

EMBODIED COGNITION

If mind and body are one, we can do more than change the body by changing the mind; we can change the mind by changing the body. And while the large psychological effects of physical changes such as illness and activity like exercise are obvious, these effects can also happen on a very small scale.

One example of mind-body unity involving studies of embodied cognition comes from John Bargh's psychology laboratory at Yale.[19] He and Lawrence Williams conducted a simple but elegant study. Research participants were asked to hold either a cup of hot coffee or a glass of iced coffee. They were then handed a questionnaire that asked for impressions about a person described on the form. Those participants who a moment before held hot coffee saw the described person as warmer than those who'd held the iced coffee. Although other researchers were subsequently unable to replicate this (the effects may be real, but only true in certain contexts), psychologists Hans Ijzerman and Gün Semin later found that holding a warm drink led people to feel closer to those they were asked to think about than when holding a cold beverage.[20]

People also tend to be happier and more satisfied with their lives when the weather is warm. Psychologist Naomi Eisenberger found that when our body temperature is up, we feel more connected to people than when our temperature is low.[21] Perhaps even more interesting is her work on social rejection. Participants in a virtual ball-tossing game who were not thrown the ball felt socially rejected.[22] Using fMRI data, she found that the brain patterns of rejection in the anterior cingulate cortex are the same as those of physical pain. If, as Eisenberger believes, physical and psychological pain patterns are found in the same part of the brain, the implication would be that physical pain could be ameliorated by psychological means.

One of my favorite experiments on this was conducted by the psychologists Fritz Strack and Sabine Stepper of the University of Würzburg in Germany, and Leonard Martin of the University of North Carolina at Greensboro.[23] Participants who had no idea of the purpose of the study were told to hold a pencil either with their lips or between their teeth. The former action affects the same muscles as a frown, while the latter mimics a smile. Participants were then asked to rate cartoons for how amusing they were. Those whose bodies were surreptitiously forced to frown were less amused than those unintentionally smiling. I have fun when telling my students about this study—I put a pencil between my teeth half the time and then between my lips for the rest of the storytelling. But more important than my own amusement, the results make clear that changing the body simultaneously changes the mind.

THE MIND AND THE SENSES

Seeing the body as separate from the mind encourages the belief in set limits for our senses. In discussing how vision can vary, I often ask the audience how much more quickly they spot a favorite restaurant when they are hungry than when they are not. Research my lab conducted with eye charts used by optometrists and ophthalmologists provided a more formal demonstration.[24] On standard eye charts, the letters get progressively smaller from top to bottom. As such, they create the expectation that at some point we will not be able to see the letters at the very bottom. In one study I alluded to earlier, we reversed the chart, putting the largest type at the bottom and thereby reversing the expectation. Sure enough, we found that now people could read lines that they couldn't before.

We tried another experiment, based on people's expectation that about two-thirds of the way down the standard eye chart they wouldn't be able to read the letters. We asked them to look at a chart that began a third of the way down from the original chart. When they started out by reading letters that were much smaller than on the standard chart, people could see letters that they couldn't see before.

Probably by necessity, the medical world can work only with normative and probabilistic information based on large numbers of people. Nevertheless, there is room for improvement in how this information is communicated to us as individuals. Imagine that instead of being told your vision was 20/60, you were told that according to this particular test *right now,* your vision measured 20/60. Based on my experiments and my belief in the power of the mind-body, I bet that with just that small linguistic change, performance would improve for at least a subset of people the next time they take an eye exam.

The ability to perceive changes in our senses came home to me personally when I had a problem with a contact lens. I wore the lens in my left eye for reading. One night I tried to remove it before going to bed. As my fingers struggled to find it, I almost scratched my eye. Fortunately, before doing serious harm, I realized I'd forgotten to put it in in the first place. Upon reflection, I realized that my vision had been fine all day. Trying to practice what I preach, I decided to leave the lens out again the next day and see what happened. That was over four years ago, and I still don't need glasses to read.

I've since done research on whether sensory abilities need to be "fixed." Karyn Gunnet-Shoval and I tested the hearing of 103 college students.[25] The participants were told that we were interested in individual differences in sensory and information processing. We divided the students into four groups. All had their hearing tested and were then asked to listen to a podcast of their choice. One group was told that we expected that listening to the podcast would lead to an improvement in their hearing in later tests. The next group was simply asked to listen to the podcast. A third group was told that having their hearing artificially improved by listening to the podcast at a low volume could help improve their hearing afterward. The fourth group was asked to listen to the podcast, set at a lower volume for the full thirty minutes, but given no expectations. Thus, participants either expected improvement or not, and listened either at a normal or below normal volume.

The results of the tests showed that listening to a podcast

at a very low volume, with or without expectations for improvement, led to hearing scores that were higher than on the initial tests. As with the vision studies, making the task harder did indeed make it easier at the next attempt.

IMAGINED EATING

As an undergraduate, I read an article for my psychophysics class that had a lasting influence on me. It was by an early American psychologist named Mary Cheves West Perky and was written in 1910.[26] Perky considered real experience versus imagined experience and essentially found no difference between the two. In her study, as I recall, participants stared at a screen and were to imagine various items like a banana or a tomato. At some point, without the participants knowing, an image—of a banana, for example—appeared on the screen. When questioned later, they thought they had imagined it. Thinking about this more recently, I find it hard to believe that the brain is wired to differentiate between the two—real versus imagined—since our beliefs influence our perceptions all the time. We may look at the same thing in different contexts and see different things. If real and imagined experiences can have the same effects, then all sorts of possibilities open up to us.

In my early teens, I spent Saturdays with my friend Lois. She was a few years older than I was and always chose what we'd do for the day. I was happy just to go along. We'd often go out for ice cream. Since I was always watching my weight while she didn't have to, I would simply sit with her while she made her way through a banana split or a hot fudge sundae. I would imagine myself eating each spoonful as it left the dish and found its way into her mouth. Funny enough, when we left the table, both of us felt full. Many years later, I came upon a research study by Carey Morewedge and colleagues in which people were asked to imagine eating cheese.[27] Some were asked to imagine eating it many times, others imagined eating it fewer times. Those who imagined eating it many times consumed less when offered actual cheese. They were full from the imagined ingestion. Although not an experiment, perhaps the most dramatic example of the impact of imagined eating comes from the work of my former Harvard colleague Lenore Weitzman and her coauthor Dalia Ofer of the Hebrew University of Jerusalem.[28]

Drawing on memoirs and interviews with Jews who survived the Holocaust, Weitzman and Ofer write about the overwhelming obsession with hunger among both men and women in the concentration camps. However, while both sexes faced and suffered from systematic starvation, they found that women were more likely to engage in behavior that seemed to help them cope. At night, after a long day of hard labor, they would often gather in their barracks and talk about food—especially the food they had eaten on Jewish holidays and the elaborate menus they had prepared for weddings and bar mitzvahs. They also recalled—and debated—the best way to make well-known Jewish foods such as challah (bread for the Jewish Sabbath) and had endless discussions about the most sumptuous desserts. As one woman said, "I learned to cook in Auschwitz; by the time I was liberated I knew many recipes for desserts, especially for Palacsinta (a Hungarian crepes dessert), by heart."

Weitzman and Ofer write that the women somehow seemed to feel satiated by recalling the tastes of these special foods. If this were not the case, and thinking about food made them hungrier, it's hard to imagine that people who were starving would engage in these thoughts.

The women also talked as if the memories of their former lives helped them transcend, if only momentarily, their harsh surroundings and humiliation in the camp. Remembering those happy meals of the past also allowed them to imagine a future in which they would once again cook for their families, and believing that they had a future gave them strength.

While Weitzman and Ofer are careful to remind us of the real-world consequences of starvation in the camps, they note that women in some camps actually wrote cookbooks (such as *In Memory's Kitchen*, written in Theresienstadt) as a testament to the importance of talking about food and sharing recipes in helping them survive and affirm they had a future.[29]

Perhaps other appetites can also be satisfied virtually. When *Mad Men* was first on TV, everyone on the program smoked. When smokers see someone light up, they often want to have a cigarette themselves. I once turned on the program in the middle of an episode, and someone had just put a cigarette out. I wondered if just seeing a cigarette primes the desire, or if imagining smoking leads people to light up. If the latter, then seeing someone put out a cigarette won't lead to lighting one up. I also wondered whether imagining smoking a full cigarette, like my imagined eating, could be satisfying in itself, without actually lighting up. As of this writing, I'm in the process of testing the hypothesis.

IMAGINARY EXERCISE

In an intriguing study of mental exercise by Vinoth Ranganathan and colleagues, participants who either mentally exercised a finger or mentally flexed their elbows over three months were compared to two control groups: a group who physically did the exercises and one who did neither.[30] The results were striking. Compared to the no-activity group, the group that did the physical exercise increased their finger strength by 53 percent; and the group that did the mental exercise improved by 35 percent. There's no way to know how much of the imagined exercise was actually performed, which may account for the difference between imagined and real. Regardless, the results are remarkable.

The effects of imaginary exercise have been shown in other studies as well. For example, just thinking about playing a sport can improve performance.[31] One study showed that a hip exercise program consisting entirely of mental imagery was as effective as actual physical exercise. Hip muscle strength increased 23.7 percent versus 28.3 percent, which are statistically equivalent results.[32] A no-treatment control group showed no improvement. A member of my lab, Francesco Pagnini, asked female volleyball players to imagine that they were flying for five minutes.[33] They significantly improved their jump heights, compared to a control group who simply watched an unrelated video.

The concept of mind-body unity can also reduce symptoms. In one study, our lab asked people with arthritis to watch a two-minute video of the hands of a performing pianist every day for ten straight days.[34] While watching the video, participants either mindfully imagined playing the piano (mental simulation), mindfully noticed aspects of the music (mindful listening), or simply listened to the music to relax. Self-reported measures of arthritis symptoms, as well as physiological measures of strength, dexterity, and flexibility, were taken before and after the treatment. While relaxation did not lead to improvements, the mindful imaginary playing and the mindful listening treatments both led to improvements on self-reported pain and physiological measures of dexterity and wrist and finger flexibility.

INTERESTING POSSIBILITIES

There are many other interesting hypotheses that mind-body unity theory suggests. One of them concerns plastic surgery. What happens when a person gets a facelift? Does the person now believe he or she looks younger, even if by objective standards they do not? I believe that if they embrace their new self, very possibly yes. Mind-body unity would not be the only thing at work, of course. People might treat you as if you're younger, too, and that could result in other positive effects.

Breast cancer is typically associated with women and not men. What would happen if a woman imagined herself in a man's body? Could this reduce a tumor in her breast? This might not be as far-fetched as it sounds. There is already research showing that transgender men (female sex assigned at birth, male gender identity) had a lower risk of breast cancer than the general female population.[35] This becomes even more interesting when we consider that these people are taking hormones, and hormone replacement therapy can increase the risk of breast cancer.

An alternative explanation to the mind-body unity hypothesis is that people who feel trapped in a woman's body have more testosterone than most women to start, and since testosterone protects against breast cancer, they are less likely to have it.

An interesting study that supports the mind-body unity explanation for why transgender men are less likely to get breast cancer looked at the act of firing someone, which, because it is generally considered to be easier for men, may be seen as a masculine behavior.[36] The researchers found that when women and men pretended to fire someone, their testosterone increased. Thus, just acting like a man may stimulate testosterone and thereby add protection against breast cancer.

All of this research makes clear to me the possibilities that are opened up by understanding the unity of mind and body.

CHAPTER 7

Placebos and Outliers

But still try, for who knows what is possible?
—MICHAEL FARADAY

My ideas about mind-body unity take on new dimensions when we consider the body of research on placebos. Most of us know placebos as harmless sugar pills used in research where one group gets the real medication and the comparison group gets the placebo to see if the medication will outperform the sugar pill. In the distant past, other inert substances were used to bring about cures. In 1794, Ranieri Gerbi rubbed worm secretions on his patients' aching teeth, and the pain vanished for more than 60 percent of them for an entire year.[1] At various times in history, dried fox lungs, the eyes of toads, mercury, leeches, and electric current were all effective cures. Thomas Jefferson wrote about how his doctor, a prominent physician, often gave people placebos and believed disease was largely psychological.[2] Perhaps the most famous American physician of the early twentieth century, Richard Cabot, remarked, "I was brought up, as I suppose every physician is, to use placebos . . . for acting upon a patient's symptoms through his mind."[3]

Many other "treatments" we now consider bizarre have also functioned as placebos. Franz Mesmer was a physician in the early 1800s who believed energy could be transferred between animate and inanimate objects.[4] Following in his footsteps, mesmerists used magnets, touch, and magnetized water to heal people, ostensibly by "correcting imbalances." The most egregious case I've found in the literature was one in which pressure was applied to a woman's vagina with a magnet until she "convulsed," which was taken as evidence of the treatment's effectiveness. In a 1784 study, mesmerism was "scientifically" investigated. A tree was magnetized, and patients were told they'd be treated by standing in front of it. But patients were taken to a different tree and still got better. Their beliefs, and not magnetism, were the true cause of their healing. I wonder which of the treatments we currently use will sound as strange to those reading about them in the future as these do to us today.

There are two things to be especially careful with concerning placebos. The first is to make sure that they are harmless. Standing in front of a non-magnetized tree is quite different from covering your body with leeches. The other concerns attributions of causality. We must remember that placebos are simply a prod for the mind to heal the body—or, as we might better put it, for the mind-body to heal. Too often, the irrelevant placebo itself is given credit. For example, homeopathy employs extremely diluted mixtures of natural substances to cure diseases. The mixtures are diluted by factors of trillions upon trillions of times. This is fine, and in fact may even be better than a sugar pill as a placebo, because sugar could cause some physical reactions whereas homeopathy is indistinguishable from drinking water. If a homeopathic treatment works, however, we should be careful to give credit to the patient, and not the drink. It is the human body that is bringing about the cure.

If we don't keep these caveats in mind, we might get stuck in a mindless causal loop: Did the homeopathic treatment work? Great, that's proof that homeopathy works. Did the homeopathic treatment not work? That's probably because we didn't use enough of it, so we should increase the dose.

This may be relatively harmless in the case of drinking water, but the exact same logic applied to leeches, which means we may end up putting too many leeches on too many people. In both cases, if things don't get better, it might be time to mindfully look for additional alternatives to explore rather than mindlessly continue trying the same failed thing. In his book *Black Box Thinking*, Matthew Syed refers to this kind of more-leeches thinking as "closed-loop thinking," a sad, mindless process in which no amount of data or evidence can ever lead to any new conclusion.[5]

PLACEBO POWER

Whether people are given sugar pills, saline injections, or sham surgery, when someone believes the treatment will provide a cure, a cure often follows. Among the more striking examples is one in which the patient was told ipecac would stop vomiting and it did stop vomiting, even though ipecac is a medication that *induces* vomiting.[6] Many patients who receive antibiotics for a viral sore throat get better. But antibiotics—powerful against bacterial infections—actually have no known medical effect on viral infections. And the psychiatrist Irving Kirsch did an interesting study showing that people get the "jitters" from caffeine only when they consume caffeine *and* know that they consumed it.[7]

We also know that the more arduous the treatment, the more likely it will be effective. Thus, sham surgery is more effective than injections, which are more effective than pills. The sham surgery data are amazing. In 1959, Leonard Cobb, a cardiologist, followed patients who were scheduled to have an internal mammary artery ligation, a procedure that constricts blood vessels to reduce chest pain.[8] He found that patients who actually had the procedure did no better or worse than patients who underwent a sham procedure. Both reported immediate relief from chest pain, and in both cases the relief lasted at least three months.

Studies have also tested whether sham surgery is as good as traditional surgery. (Participants all signed consent forms informing them that they might be in the placebo group.) One of these studies looked at the efficacy of intracranial fetal neural cells implantation for people with Parkinson's disease.[9] Patients in the sham surgery group were given anesthesia and the surgeon drilled a hole in their heads so that the patients felt as though the "surgery" was real, but did not receive the neural cell implant. The benefits were as good as with actual surgery. In another of these studies, knee surgery was compared with sham surgery in which incisions are made but no actual procedure is carried out.[10] The arthroscopic surgeries were no more effective than the sham surgery. Patients were tested for two years for pain and how well they could walk.

While few of us have had to deal with these sorts of surgeries or procedures, the findings regarding the effectiveness of less invasive placebos are numerous. In one study, warts were painted with bright colors and patients were told they would disappear when the color wore off.[11] They did. Asthmatics were told they were inhaling a bronchodilator that would increase dilation in the airways, and significant relief followed, even though they were using an inhaler without any active drug.[12] Patients with pain from a wisdom tooth extraction who were treated with a fake ultrasound application experienced as much relief as from a real one.[13] Fifty-two percent of colitis patients treated with a placebo reported feeling better; in 50 percent of the patients the inflamed intestines looked better via sigmoidoscopy thereafter as well.[14]

Behavioral economist Dan Ariely and his colleagues found that the more we pay for pills, the more effective they tend to be.[15] Let's think about that for a moment. If two people take the exact same medication but with different costs (or if one person takes an expensive pill on one occasion and the same pill costing less on another), what accounts for the differences in health? Somehow, their expectations for improvement based on how much the treatment cost translated into measurable improvement. So, if you're the one making yourself better, you might ask, why bother with medications at all? Perhaps it's because we've come to rely on medications and medical treatments and don't often give ourselves a chance to get better without them.

In another study, students were asked to keep track of their colds, the medication they took for relief, and its effectiveness. Those who paid the list price for their cold meds, rather than a discounted price, got better faster.[16] In another study these same researchers found that students who drank a higher priced energy drink felt less fatigue and performed a cognitive anagram task better.[17] This raises a moral issue. I don't think the answer to better health is higher prices. What is important about these findings is the support for the idea that our beliefs are essential to our health.

We even have expectations regarding the color of the pills we take. Research has found that yellow is most effective for depression;[18] green is good for anxiety; white is good for ulcers even if they contain only lactose (which is not effective for treating ulcers); and red pills are good for energy.[19]

Certain words can act as a placebo, too: Their power may be a pill so simple that it's not hard to swallow. Just as placebos are conditioned to physical responses, words often occasion behavioral or attitudinal responses mindlessly. In some of my earliest research, it turned out the simple word "because" persuaded people to act even if it was not accompanied by any new information.[20] We approached students at the front of a long line of people waiting to use a copier and asked either, "May I please use the Xerox machine?" or "May I please use the Xerox machine because I need to make copies?" Note that no particular reason to use the copier was offered. Nevertheless, many people swallowed the "because" and let us go ahead of them.

University College London math professor Alan Sokal tested the power of language in a similar way.[21] He submitted a nonsensical paper to an academic journal that proposed that quantum gravity was a social and linguistic construct. Since words like "quantum gravity" have an air of importance, they are often accepted without question. Sokal's paper was accepted for publication because, in his words, "It was liberally salted with nonsense that a) sounded good and b) flattered the editors' ideological preconceptions."

Then there are what have come to be known as the "grievance studies" conducted by philosopher Peter Boghossian, mathematician James Lindsay, and author and British cultural critic Helen Pluckrose.[22] They wrote and submitted for academic publication twenty articles about things that on their face would seem outrageous: dogs engaging in rape culture; rewriting Hitler's *Mein Kampf* in feminist language, and so on. Their aim was to show that a lack of academic rigor had developed in journal publishing and that even absurd topics could see the light of day when they come from people with good credentials. Astonishingly, only six of their articles were rejected. Four were published, three more were accepted and prepared for publication, and seven were still under review when the hoax was revealed. When it comes to pills and words, we have strong expectations. As Paul Simon sang, "A man hears what he wants to hear and disregards the rest."

STRONG MEDICINE

To bring a drug to market, pharmaceutical companies must show in research that the drug is *more* effective than a placebo when tested in a randomized controlled clinical trial. What many people don't realize is that there are countless studies in which the placebo is as effective as or even outperforms the drug. These studies are not accepted for publication, which is why we never hear about them. What we should learn from these studies is not that a particular drug is ineffective but rather how effective the placebo may have been, especially since drugs often have side effects, and placebos typically don't. I believe this makes placebos our *most* effective medicine.

If a research participant expects side effects and doesn't experience them, they may conclude they were in the placebo group and thus not expect or experience improvements. If participants in the real drug group experience side effects, they may conclude they are in the real drug group and hence expect the drug to work. The bigger the side effects, the stronger the belief that the person is in the drug group. As a result, even when the drug outperforms the placebo, it may be a function of beliefs.

A 2009 study recounted the experience of a patient who had cancerous tumors the size of oranges in his armpits, groin, chest, and abdomen.[23] His doctors believed that he had fewer than two weeks to live. Then he was given a new experimental drug and the tumors vanished. When the drug was later declared ineffective in a trial and he was told about the trial results, his tumors reappeared. Then the patient was given what was described to him as a "double-strength" medication—which was actually a placebo—and the tumors disappeared again. He had been symptom-free for two months when he read that this drug, too, was worthless. He died a few days later.

I also believe that some clinical trial outcomes are positive because they encourage people to notice symptom variability. We take a drug, we expect it to have an effect, and we notice subtle differences in how we feel. Because all symptoms vary, there will often be moments of improvement, and these observations may increase our belief in the efficacy of the drug. Research with antidepressants supports this view, in that the more likely it is that people know something about placebo research, the more the effect of the placebo is magnified in them. They look for improvements and they find them.[24] Moreover, there is evidence that actual drugs work best in individuals who exhibit strong placebo effects. More on this in the next chapter.

Still, much of the lay public often mistakenly think of placebos as ineffective. But many of these same people believe strongly in neuroscience because, their logic goes, if you can show something is happening in the brain, it must be real. But research is revealing that the brain responds the same way to placebos as it does to drugs. As doctor and author Jerome Groopman writes, "It may be that the more we discover about the brain, the easier it will be to disregard the apparent divide between mind and body."

Neuroscientist Tor Wager and colleagues at Dartmouth College looked at what happens in the brain when we unknowingly take placebos.[25] Using functional magnetic resonance imaging (fMRI), they found that a placebo analgesic reduced brain activity in "pain sensitive areas of the brain (thalamus, insula, anterior cingulate cortex) and anticipation of pain was associated with increased activity in the prefrontal cortex." It may be that certain genetic predispositions encourage different responses in us, but I believe the placebo effect is available to us all. If you agree that anything happening on any level of the mindful body is happening on every level, it stands to reason that researchers seeking evidence of the placebo effect in different parts of the brain are likely to find it.

WHO DO YOU BELIEVE?

The other day my tennis game was off. I asked the pro if my racket needed to be restrung. She asked me when I last had it restrung. I had no idea, and so we decided it was a smart thing to do now. The next time I played with my newly strung racket, my game was as good as or better than ever. Was it because of the racket or because my expectations brought more focus to my game? If the latter, I was in control of my play. If the former, the racket was in charge.

This is the same story with placebos. Unbeknownst to us, many of us are given placebos to help us heal. If we attribute the reduction in symptoms or cure to the prescribed pill when it was a placebo, we stay dependent on the medication. How much better off might we be if we were told the medication was a placebo? Would we try to take more control of our health the next time the symptoms appeared?

Although doctors are loath to tell us that they have prescribed placebos to us, perhaps this unwritten policy should be called into question. Regardless of what I know, if I am ill and take a pill and recover—and it was due to the placebo effect—who cured me? Clearly if the pill was inert, I must have cured myself. If the doctor had told me this and made me realize that I healed myself, would I be more likely to be able to control my health in the future? The doctor probably doesn't tell me it was a placebo because she believes that doing so would cast doubt over the next prescription she writes. It's a trade-off: Tell me it was a placebo to increase my control over my health versus running the risk that I'll no longer believe in the efficacy of medicine. Put another way, is it better to increase my belief in myself or my belief in the pill?

There is a growing body of research on the "open-label placebo." Indeed, as early as 1965, researchers examined the effects of giving a placebo to people who knew it was a placebo.[26] They found that the transparency didn't render the pill ineffective. That is, taking a placebo and knowing it is a placebo may still reduce symptoms. More recently, the open-label placebo was tested with cancer survivors.[27] In some cases, the cancer was gone but fatigue still lingered. Other scientists looked at the effects of a placebo compared to treatment in cancer survivors still experiencing fatigue.[28] For three weeks, some participants received a pill labeled as a placebo while others received their treatment as usual. Despite being labeled as a placebo, the pills still had a positive effect. I believe this shows that as long as patients are induced to have positive expectations, an open-label placebo approach should work.

SPONTANEOUS REMISSIONS

Again, as I described in the introduction, my mother's experience with cancer left me with many unanswered questions. When she found a lump under her arm, the medical world took over. They scheduled a biopsy to see if the primary site was in her breast. I asked them what the course of action would be if it were. They said they'd do a radical mastectomy. I asked what the next step would be if the breast were not the primary site. They said they would do a radical mastectomy. If they were planning a mastectomy in either case, then why put her through another biopsy? I was still young, so all I did was ask annoying questions without having much influence over the situation.

She had the surgery and went home for some time, but subsequent CT scans revealed more cancer. At this point despite my belief in the importance of perceived control, I took control over her life. I tried to keep anyone who felt sorry for her or who was pessimistic from visiting her. I shared stories of people who made amazing recoveries, and even asked one of these people who was in the hospital for a checkup to pay her a visit. The woman told her that the doctors had said she had only six months to live. Thinking this was true, the woman spent almost all her money. Eighteen months later she was alive but without the funds to help her enjoy it.

When my mother went through chemo, she was nauseated, her hair fell out, and it seemed that it was all for nothing. The next series of scans showed that the cancer had spread to her pancreas. The doctors told her she had only a few more months to live.

Then her cancer vanished. There was no trace of it on the scans. It just disappeared. It was a spontaneous remission.

As this was just a sample of one—without a comparison group—there was and is no way to be sure how to explain what happened to her. I've been interested in spontaneous remissions ever since.

Spontaneous remissions do happen, and the medical world has no great explanation for them. You might think that when there is a spontaneous remission, this would help shed the cancer label since the person is now cancer-free. But sadly, I think not. Hopefully today's doctors no longer utter "It'll be back" out loud after a spontaneous remission (as they did in my mother's case), but it would be hard for them not to think it. From their experience, they see patients whose spontaneous remissions reverse and the disease returns. They rarely see the ones who are permanently cured, so it is reasonable for them to infer that most spontaneous remissions will ultimately fail. But we do not know if most succeed or most fail.

From the perspective of the patient, however, the moment they find out they have improved is an important and delicate one. Perhaps there are ways doctors can be trained to deliver this wonderful news in a sustainable and mindful way. Calling it a miracle or an unexplained phenomenon and suggesting scheduled follow-ups subtly drops a mindless and pessimistic shroud over what should be ecstatic proceedings. Instead, what if doctors in such situations reminded patients about the power of the mind, that there is mind-body unity, and that, while there is still much ongoing research and many things that are still unknown about how cancer works, spontaneous and permanent remissions do indeed happen, when a patient becomes fully clear and healthy with no more need for monitoring than another similarly healthy person. "Please send me a holiday card every year" or "You are good to go now, but I will miss seeing you, so how about giving me a call to say hello in two months?" might be far superior discharge instructions than "Let's keep checking your bloodwork every month."

When healing takes place without medical intervention it is undoubtedly a puzzle for the medical world. Instances of spontaneous remission, however, provide further evidence for mind-body unity: When our minds fully believe we are well, concomitant changes in the body may become evident. It's very hard to put doubts aside, however, after being diagnosed with a dread disease.

"Science often ignores cases of spontaneous remission because it is busy looking for statistical averages," says James Gordon, MD, professor of medicine at Georgetown Medical School. "This is not good science, just convenient science. Even if they hardly ever happen, these 'miracles' are the kinds of exceptions to the ruling paradigm and inevitably create new areas of study."[29]

While spontaneous remissions may seem to be well outside the normal occurrence, I'm not sure how infrequent they actually are. After all, since many people do not go to doctors when they are sick, there is no way of knowing how many of them experience spontaneous remissions from diseases they did not even know they had. Moreover, we all know of people with diseases who lived many years beyond what was expected. I would imagine that a fair number of these people have not called their doctors to report that they are still alive, so their numbers may not be included in formal medical statistics.

Drs. Gary Challis of Carleton University and Henderikus Stam of the University of Calgary reviewed cases of spontaneous remissions and concluded that while there is little data to explain their occurrence, behavioral patterns and anecdotal evidence about the survivors' beliefs play a part.[30] Kelly Ann Turner, a researcher from the University of California at Berkeley, interviewed people from eleven countries and found similar patterns of behavior, among them being more positive, trusting, spiritual, and taking vitamins.[31] Of course, we don't know if these characteristics were a response to survival or if the attributes had a role in it. Other researchers have found that many cancer survivors believe in a higher power that could heal the body, suggesting that our thoughts matter and affect our bodies.

Once we get a diagnosis of cancer it's hard to believe we are healthy. Nevertheless, from 1978, when my mother's cancer disappeared, to this day, I have believed that if our minds are fully healthy, so too will be our bodies. Thus, to my mind, psychology might be able to provide the answer to the spontaneous remission puzzle. Time and research will tell. At this point, though, it's safe to say that as long as such beliefs do not make us refuse medical care, their downsides are minimal—except for one possibility.

If I am right and our minds have more control over our health than most people imagine, does that mean that people who succumbed to ill health and disease are to blame for their conditions? Of course not. But if at virtually every turn, the culture we are born into teaches us that our minds and bodies are separate entities, it is not surprising that we believe it. It is no different from when schools teach us things that turn out to be wrong. People are not to blame for believing that 1 + 1 always equals 2, if that is what they have been taught. Yet one cloud plus one cloud equals one cloud; one pile of laundry plus one pile of laundry equals one pile of laundry; one wad of chewing gum plus one wad of chewing gum equals one wad of chewing gum, and so on. Thus, 1 + 1 does not always equal 2. Indeed, if we are using a base 2 number system and not a base 10 number system, 1 + 1 is written as 10. As research results on mind-body unity coming from our lab and that of other labs accumulates, at some point we all may be taught how to create the mindful body. Nevertheless, we can take advantage of these findings right now and be healthier for it.

EMBODYING THE MIND

I started reading about the psychology of stress as an undergraduate and have come to believe that it is likely a bigger killer than even heart disease and cancer. With each health study I've conducted, I have become more convinced of its damaging effects.

To pursue studies on the effects of stress on disease, I started by calling some leading oncologists. Several were intrigued with the question of whether a measurement of how stressed a person was could predict the course of a disease. If we knew the stress level of people who had just been informed they had cancer, for instance, would that stress response suggest more about the course of the disease and ultimate likelihood of morbidity than the initial diagnosis?

It was easy to see that it would be difficult to gather the data for such a study. And each physician, after agreeing that I might be right, listed all the likely problems. When people first find out they have some dread disease, they're not likely to want to be in a study. Down the road, matching patients to make sure everything but the degree of stress present is the same would also be hard. As each disease progresses, stress levels change. Even if a study could be designed, who would fund it? Sources that fund medical research might see the work as psychological and outside of their purview. Similarly, funders of research in psychology likely would see the research as outside their areas of interest. Every year, however, people studying specific diseases come to the same conclusions about the effect of stress on the particular disease of their interest. Meanwhile, the role of stress is becoming even clearer and, like many once radical ideas, may eventually be seen as too obvious to test.

But mind-body unity speaks to more than just the negative effect of stress on our health. My students and I were able to conduct several studies concerning diabetes, immune functioning, and various chronic diseases to test the mind-body unity hypothesis.[32] We enlisted people with type 2 diabetes to participate in a study purportedly about the effects of diabetes on cognitive functioning. After we tested their blood glucose levels, participants played simple video games while viewing a clock on the desk and were asked to switch to a new game every fifteen minutes or so to ensure they would look at the clock.

People who have type 2 diabetes know that their blood sugar levels vary every few hours based on their biology. Rarely, if ever, do they believe it could vary based on their beliefs. Nevertheless, I believed it would. The idea came to me when I ate my first Krispy Kreme doughnut back in 2002. If you look at a doughnut and smell it and imagine eating it—everything but actually consuming it—would your blood sugar rise? Finally, I had the chance to find out. The participants in our study were randomly assigned to one of three conditions: For one group the clock in front of them was on real time; for another group the clock ran twice as fast as real time; and for the last group the clock ran half as fast as real time. The question we were investigating was whether blood sugar levels followed real or perceived time. Post-task measures revealed that perceived time was more important than real time. Other measures ruled out stress or enjoyment as alternative explanations.

In a second study, we examined the impact of psychological components on diabetic metabolism, again, a physiological process widely believed to be immune to the idiosyncrasies of subjective cognition. Specifically, we tested whether differences in the perceived amount of sugar consumption have an effect on blood glucose level in people with type 2 diabetes. Our hypothesis was that the perceived amount of sugar consumption would have an influence over blood glucose level, even when the actual amount consumed remained the same. People with type 2 diabetes were invited to taste beverages on two occasions, three days apart. We made sure that they checked the nutritional label on the beverages, which we changed from session to session, even though the actual contents of the two beverages were identical throughout the study. When we measured blood glucose levels before and after the consumption of these beverages, to track how they had changed, we found that they reflected perceived—rather than actual—sugar consumption. When a drink's label indicated high sugar content, people's blood sugar spiked after they drank it.

Broccoli has been shown to help promote insulin sensitivity and reduce blood sugar levels in people with type 2 diabetes. Think of Pavlov's dogs, who would salivate at just the sight or smell of meat once it had been repeatedly paired with ingesting the meat. If you smelled broccoli first every time you ate it, I think you could get a conditioned response to the smell. If so, just smelling broccoli could reduce blood sugar level and thus help the person with type 2 diabetes. Eventually, just imagining consuming broccoli might have the same effect. All sorts of possibilities come to mind once we recognize mind-body unity.

Many of us may know that the perception of scent (olfaction) is 85 percent of flavor perception. When we have a stuffy nose, food simply loses some of its appeal. Not surprisingly, there are clinical trial findings pointing to the ways scent can raise appetite, suppress appetite, and alter food cravings. It would seem, then, that smell provides an opportunity for satiety and weight loss. Smell a croissant first and you will want to eat more of it. Smell chocolate and, again, you'll want to eat more of it. On the other hand, if we smell steak before eating either the croissant or chocolate, we would probably eat less. This suggests interesting ways we can use smell to control our weight. But weight is not the only thing that can change by mindfully using the power of smell.

Proust was onto something even bigger than he knew when he ate a crumb of a madeleine soaked in his aunt's concoction of lime flowers and his mind was flooded with memories. Smells and tastes from the past make the past lively and thus may aid in the counterclockwise effect described earlier.

More support for mind-body unity comes from a study conducted by Alia Crum and her colleagues.[33] It must have been a fun study to be in since participants were all given milkshakes to drink. Some of them, however, were led to think the milkshake was high in calories (620 calories to be exact) and some that it was "lite" (only 140 calories), despite the fact that it was the same in both conditions. The researchers measured ghrelin, which is known as the hunger hormone. It's produced in the stomach and is highest before meals, when we tend to be hungry. Thinking they had consumed the very fattening milkshake led to a steep drop in ghrelin, which was consistent with the degree to which they felt full.

In one of our most recent studies, my graduate student Peter Aungle led members of our lab to look at wound healing as a function of perceived versus real time.[34] Rightly so, the institutional review board would not be happy with us harming people with big wounds to test our hypothesis. Therefore, we recruited people to be in a study assessing the effectiveness of Chinese cupping therapy, a process wherein suction cups are placed on parts of the body to increase blood flow to the area to help cell repair, decrease pain, and increase chi, or life force. The cupping leaves a circular bruise in the spot where it was placed. Our purpose, however, was simply to create a minor "wound" and see how fast it healed as a function of expectations. Participants were asked to monitor the wound every few minutes. Each participant went through three sessions. In one session the clock they watched was rigged so that it ran twice as fast as real time. In another session the clock ran half as fast as real time. And for another session the clock displayed real time. The order in which participants experienced the different clock times was systematically varied. Would wound healing follow real or perceived time? The wounds indeed healed based on perceived rather than real time. That is, compared to real time, the wound healed faster when the clock ran fast and slower when it ran slow.

Another set of our ongoing studies considers immune functioning and the "nocebo effect" on common cold symptomatology and immune function.[35] A nocebo is the opposite of a placebo—expectation is that negative outcomes will follow a sham treatment. In our investigation, we wondered if expectations could lead to a cold in spite of the absence of exposure to a cold virus. We conducted two studies to test the hypothesis that just believing we have a cold without the introduction of a cold virus would increase the odds of developing cold symptoms. Two interventions were used to create a nocebo mindset: Participants were asked to act as if they had a cold and then were told they were in an early stage of having a cold. Both self-induced and primed mindsets resulted in an increase in cold symptoms and a higher rate of developing a cold at the end of the study sessions. We also observed changes in the participants' immunoglobulins, the antibodies that fight viruses and bacteria and protect our mucous membranes.

In these experiments, participants arrived at the lab, and researchers took a sample of immunoglobulin A (IgA) from their saliva. IgA levels increase in the presence of the common cold virus, so we knew these levels would show us whether the treatments were successful in inducing a cold. We also assessed cold symptoms using the common cold questionnaire, which assesses symptoms across four domains: general symptoms, nasal symptoms, throat symptoms, and chest symptoms. Half of the participants were asked to think of themselves as having a cold and to imagine the symptoms while they were surrounded by cold-relevant stimuli like tissues, chicken soup, and Vaseline. These participants also watched a video of people coughing and sneezing.

The comparison group was given the same questionnaire as the experimental group, but these participants watched a neutral video about knitting. Six days later, we called the participants in both groups and asked them whether they had a cold. Thirty-eight percent of those primed to have a cold had developed a cold, versus only 5 percent of the comparison group.

Being told you have a cold is a relatively passive situation, even if it is by someone you believe to be a physician. What happens if you instead actively imagine the condition of having a cold? On the one hand, you lose the passive belief and trustworthiness of a doctor telling you you have a cold; on the other hand, it is a more active mental process. Which is more convincing? We found that it was the latter: Actively imagining a cold led to significantly more cold-like symptoms. In other words, an active imagination is more immediately powerful than accepting passive external information. Over time, however, the effect was different: Participants in the passive condition were more likely to report a cold a week later. Perhaps the imagination works more quickly but fades more quickly, too, while being "diagnosed" with a cold is information that rattles around in your brain for a few days, building up credibility.

Most potent of all in this early investigation was the double-barreled combination. These participants were first asked to actively imagine they had a cold, and then later informed by a "physician" that they were indeed getting a cold. In this group, self-reported colds were most prevalent. In other words, they were the ones who were most convinced they had colds. But did they? Yes—their elevated IgA levels indicated their body was indeed fighting off a cold.

All this is to say that it appears it is possible to get a cold without the introduction of a cold virus.

Of course, the cold did not necessarily appear out of nowhere—it may be that in both studies a dormant virus was primed. If participants can use their minds to activate a dormant virus, perhaps it is not far-fetched to imagine they could also block or mitigate an active one.

One might think the natural reaction to these results from a medical scholar would be amazement or skepticism about the results. What we have found, however, from reports from the doctors who reviewed our manuscript about the study's results, was just the opposite. One reviewer dismissed it as unoriginal since we had already published the diabetes paper. It was as if everyone was now convinced of mind-body unity and therefore no more research was required. They were suggesting that it was obvious that people without any exposure to a virus will experience symptoms of that virus. If so, then the opposite would seem to be true, too, and the entire industry of cold-reducing medicines would be shuttered.

As Schopenhauer is presumed to have said, "All research passes through three phases: First it is ridiculed; then it is violently opposed; and third it is accepted as self-evident." Thus, it's not just that mindsets are hard to change, but that once changed, people act as if they always knew it. The next journal editor, who did accept the manuscript, clearly hadn't reached the third stage.

Sadly, the belief in mind-body dualism is still strong. Putting psychogenic disorders like hysteria aside, the prevailing belief regarding most diseases—from the common cold to cancer—is still that to become sick there has to be the introduction of bacteria or a virus. Nevertheless, research coming out of our lab and the labs of other psychologists is bringing this view into question. Even the common cold may be a product of our thoughts.

Our mindfulness research is questioning many assumed limits to health and well-being. When we overcome passive acceptance of labels, prime positive instead of pessimistic expectations, and recognize the power of the placebo, we stretch the possibilities of both health and well-being. I think enough research has been conducted by myself and others to finally put to rest the mindless constraints that for too long have kept us from being our healthiest selves.

CHAPTER 8

Attention to Variability

When Symptoms Change but Mindsets Don't

No disease suffered by a live man can be known, for
every living person has his own peculiarities and always
has his own peculiar, personal, novel, complicated
disease, unknown to medicine.

—LEO TOLSTOY

L ife—like reality more generally—is uncertain and always changing. On some level, we know that, because
we notice the changes from good to bad (although we
don't as often notice the changes from bad to good). When it
comes to a medical diagnosis, however, we often *don't* accept
this uncertainty; without medical intervention or a doctor
telling us we're cured, we tend to presume our diagnosis will
stay the same, our symptoms will stay the same, and our reactions to those symptoms will stay the same. This is especially
the case if and when we find out we have some chronic illness.
Precisely *because* it is labeled as chronic, we mindlessly expect
that the symptoms will stay the same or perhaps get worse.

Although the changes to our health or symptoms may be

small, paying attention to them closely reveals that they are sometimes better and sometimes worse. I believe that the key to controlling our health may be in noticing these subtle changes. Indeed, noticing subtle changes and asking why they may have occurred and then testing one's hypothesis could dramatically affect all diseases. If we just assume that things will stay the same or only get worse, we give up an opportunity to see whether we have this kind of control over our bodies.

Consider this simple question: If you have been diagnosed with some disease but then don't have the attending symptoms at some point in the day, do you still have the disease? We go to the doctor's office at a single point in time. The information that is collected during this visit—cholesterol level, vision, blood pressure, pain level, pulse, and so on—is noted in our files as a snapshot of our health, that we presented with *on the day of the appointment.* These levels and health indicators are not static—they fluctuate throughout the day, week, and months. But we're typically blind to these fluctuations, mindlessly treating these numbers as fixed or baseline. Once we are given a diagnosis, the same thing happens. We tend to treat our symptoms as fixed, when surely they change continually. Sometimes the pain is greater, sometimes it is less. Getting back to that simple question: In the absence of symptoms, aren't we healthy?

When I lecture on these ideas, I sometimes ask the audience if anyone knows their cholesterol level. Someone proud of their numbers quickly raises their hand and states the number when I ask for it. Then I ask when that number was collected. Typically, people report at least six months ago, but even if they were to say "yesterday," I'd continue with my questioning: "And you haven't eaten or exercised since?" If they don't get the idea at that point, I follow up with, "If you never have it checked again, you'll die a healthy person."

On the flip side, when we *expect* to have a symptom, we tend to explain almost everything by it and remain oblivious to alternative explanations. For instance, let's say you have arthritis and so aren't surprised when you wake up with an especially sore shoulder one morning. But was the pain you experienced a function of your arthritis, or was it due to a poor night's sleep or to the fact that you sat in an awkward position while watching TV for hours the night before? There are changes you can make to avoid more shoulder pain if the source of that pain is your bed or your couch. But we assimilate to our conditions and remain blind to these potential solutions.

So, what exactly should we do? We need to notice not only when we have a symptom but when we don't have it, or have it to a different degree. We need to pay attention to the variability of our symptoms. Then we need to ask ourselves why it might be better or worse at any given moment.

ATTENTION TO VARIABILITY, UNCERTAINTY, AND MINDFULNESS

Even as medical professionals must use a certain vocabulary to shorthand the complexities of health and disease—referring to a person's cancer as stage 3 or stage 4, for example—most doctors have come to see patients as individuals; they avoid one-size-fits-all treatments whenever possible. But not only are we each different from other people in meaningful ways, we are constantly different from ourselves. Indeed, *none of us is us.* At any moment the atoms that make up our bodies are different from the moment before. In fact, every seven to ten years virtually 100 percent of the atoms in our bodies are new.

Let's briefly consider the implications of this for medication. Medications are not tested on genetic clones; some people in a test pool will be tall, some short, some heavy, some thin, or with a metabolism that is faster or slower. Even though we might each be prescribed a dose that has supposedly been calibrated with at least our body mass in mind, too often we mindlessly take the medication as if it had been tailored *just* for us. We need to tune in to our bodies with whatever we ingest and notice subtle effects. That way we can discuss with our medical team the idea of taking a bit more or less, or even to discontinue it to enhance the overall effects.

But while doctors appreciate the ways in which symptoms may be different for different people, they are less sensitive to the idea that a given symptom will vary for a single individual. Of course, if asked whether symptoms are always the same, doctors would surely answer "no," but the fact of these differences is not something they typically attend to. It would be unreasonable to expect the medical establishment to give us eye tests, take our blood pressure, pulse, temperature, or do blood workups every day, let alone every hour. Yet again, everything about us is in constant flux.

Diseases are not static, either. Our perception of their constancy is an illusion that may cost us our health. If we view ourselves over time, we see change. If we view ourselves at the microscopic level we see change. But we're less attuned to our everyday experience of minor fluctuations.

Many sensations are assumed to be symptoms. But how many times do we have to have the symptoms to qualify for the label of "illness"? Who decides? Once we accept that label, we overlook all the disconfirmations and get sucked into believing the diagnosis is not only accurate, but permanent. Paying attention to variability may reduce our tendency to presume that our aches and pains confirm our diagnosis, even when joint stiffness could be a result of gardening for too many hours, rather than arthritis.

I often pose another question to my audiences that drives this point home. I find someone who is wearing glasses and ask them when they started wearing them and whether they ever take them off and test their vision without them. Overwhelmingly, people report that their glasses were prescribed for reading, and they put them on every time they pick up something to read—regardless of how large the font or how familiar the content. People with bifocals or trifocals wear them all the time, oblivious to momentary need. I suggest to them that they should notice variations in their ability to see. Wouldn't it be better to wean themselves off these "crutches"? If they did, they might realize, for example, that their vision is less good late in the afternoon than in the morning. The alternative to glasses then could be an energy bar or a nap.

Of course, if one's vision is significantly compromised, it makes sense to wear glasses all the time. For the rest of us, the possibility of improving our vision could awaken the possibility of other changes heretofore seen as unalterable. The same is true for hearing aids, since they can be easily put in or taken out—you can experiment without the need of a physician.

Think of this mind shift as you might when taking a laxative. If one is needed once in a while, no harm done. If you took a laxative every day, however, you'd be teaching your body to wait for that aid in order to move your bowels. You would become dependent on the laxative. To my mind, it's no different than the overreliance on eyeglasses and hearing aids.

I once asked a friend about a medicine she was taking, and she told me it was an unprescribed stool softener. I asked how often she took it. She said every day. Shouldn't she consider the amount and type of food she was eating that necessitated a daily stool softener? After all, there is a meaningful difference between fruits and vegetables and cheese and popcorn. Or between consuming very little versus eating enough to satisfy a professional football player, or a regime of many liquids versus very few. Or maybe she was taking another medication that was contributing to her constipation. Could she look into changing that regimen? All of these questions take a back seat—if they get a seat at all—when we blindly follow a daily medical regimen. We need to notice when the need for a laxative arises and when it doesn't. Doctors can't do this for us. Doctors make good consultants, but we need to stay in charge.

A friend who read an early draft of this book found that applying attention to variability helped him when his doctors diagnosed him with thyroiditis with an unknown cause and told him there was essentially nothing to do. But when he paid attention to changes in his symptoms, he noticed that he felt better if he did vigorous exercise early in the day. It seemed to "burn off" some of the symptoms and made it much easier for him to cope. There is no way the doctors, no matter how well-intentioned, could have discovered the treatment that happened to work for my friend. Perhaps the morning exercise wouldn't help anyone else. That's why we have to see for ourselves. Therein lies the power of the attention-to-variability approach.

Another early reader of this book sent me her use of this attention-to-variability strategy. "I've been battling vertigo on and off for several months. Just last week I woke in the middle of the night and knew I was in its grasp again—I was spinning, sweating, trying not to vomit. I went to the doctor the next day for an 'adjustment' (essentially, they induce the sensation while trying to get your ear canal crystals to go back where they belong) and have been better since. But last night it got bad again and I lay awake for a couple of hours, white-knuckling through the worst of it. About an hour into it, I remembered your idea of noticing variability of symptoms, so I started to try to compare last night's bout with last week's and then also to compare what I was feeling in about ten-minute increments. No surprise to you, I was able to discern distinct highs and lows and to notice that last night was significantly better than last week's 'attack.' I noticed that my brain had somehow come to understand that I was not, in fact, falling or spinning and so even though my eyes said so, my stomach didn't lurch the way it did last week; my brain got the memo on that. That made me hopeful and calmer, and I eventually was able to stop the world spinning." Needless to say, this attention-to-variability treatment is available to all of us.

How often does a person have to drink to have a drinking problem, and who decides? Let's use the concept of attention to variability to an advantage here. Consider keeping a diary where every two hours you note an instance of one of four categories: You wanted a drink or you didn't want a drink, and you either had a drink or you didn't have a drink. Looking back at your journal after a week, it's most likely that each category has some entries: For example, sometimes you had a drink when you didn't even want one, and sometimes you didn't have a drink when you wished you could have. This leads to a different picture than the one many problem drinkers cling to, thinking they have no control over their alcohol consumption. What were the circumstances where you didn't want a drink, or you wanted it but denied yourself? Attention to these different situations tells us we do have control. We also begin to notice that there is no sharp distinction between "external" and "internal" variability. This leads to an awareness of how virtually everything changes: symptom and sensation intensity and durability, as well as where in the body it is occurring.

In early work we found that by noticing variability, people could learn to control their heart rate. My then students Laura Delizonna, Ryan Williams, and I asked participants to record their heart rate every day for a week, at various times depending on the condition they were in.[1] The attention-to-variability group did this every three hours and noted the activity they were engaged in at the time and whether their heart rate increased or decreased from the previous time they measured it. This made them more mindful of the variability. Everyone returned to the lab a week after the monitoring and was asked to raise or lower their heart rate without any instructions as to how to do it. The attention-to-variability group was better able to do this. Moreover, those who scored high on our mindfulness scale exercised greater control over heart rate regulation, regardless of the experimental condition to which participants had been assigned.

In another experiment, my Israeli colleague Sigal Zilcha-Mano and I tested attention-to-variability intervention on pregnancy.[2] The women who participated were given instructions to attend to the variability of their sensations (positive and negative) at weeks twenty-five to thirty of their pregnancy. We found that when pregnant women attended to the variability of the sensations they experienced, they had an easier pregnancy and, based on a number of health measures taken by their doctors—the Apgar score—they had healthier babies. The Apgar score is used by medical staff in delivery wards worldwide to quickly evaluate the clinical status of newborns one minute and five minutes after birth. It is determined by examining the infant for five criteria: heart rate, respiratory effort, muscle tone, reflex irritability, and color. Apgar scores were significantly better for the mindful groups.

When we recognize changes in sensation, intensity, and durability inside the body and external cues like the time of day, we notice more about our experiences and feelings. Which parts of our body are most or least affected? How are the sensations changing over time? How do these changes affect our behavior? By noticing these changes, we regain control over our health, and symptoms come to be experienced as less insurmountable.

A similar perspective could be applied to menopause. Do

women who are going through menopause get hot flashes all night, every night? Probably not. Attending to the variability, they may notice that the hot flashes are more intense at some times and attending to that variability could be similarly helpful. Ironically, I missed out on that advantage myself. Many years ago, I was complaining to a friend about hot flashes. She was surprised since I rarely complained about anything. She said, "If I complained about hot flashes to you, you'd tell me to consider their advantages, like burning calories." I was suddenly excited about having a new weight-loss program without having to diet. And oddly and almost sadly now, from that point forward, I never had another hot flash.

Put plainly, paying attention to variability helps us see that symptoms come and go, which helps us home in on the situations and circumstances that might contribute to these fluctuations so that we might exert some control over them. Having that kind of increased control gives rise to solutions that otherwise would not be forthcoming, as well as more optimism and less stress, which give rise to greater health in general.

Stress doesn't need to consume our thinking about our health, but it often plays a central role. If we're certain a health crisis won't arise, and then it does, we're hit over the head by it. If we're certain that illness or injury is going to happen, our fear increases with every symptom. If we're uncertain, but believe we should be certain, as when the doctor asks us how long we've been experiencing the symptom, that too increases our stress.

But there is a fourth choice, and one that allows us the kind of control I mentioned above. We need to change our thinking, where we acknowledge uncertainty but retain confidence. It is true that uncertainty can often be stressful, but by accepting change as constant, we can exploit the power of that uncertainty. If we acknowledge that no one really knows for sure—nor can anyone know because everything is always changing, and everything looks different from different perspectives—not knowing itself becomes less stressful.

What does it mean to be confident but uncertain? When we know we don't have all the answers but are willing to take action anyway, it's easier to act with confidence. Typically, people let their uncertainty get in the way of taking any action. Should I do this? Should I do that? I can't be sure, so I often do nothing. Once we acknowledge that everything is uncertain, uncertainty just becomes part and parcel of everyday life and doesn't stop us in our tracks. When we feel confident, we want to get more things done, and we're likely to be content with our accomplishments. We're also more likely to feel proud of ourselves.

When we're comfortable with being uncertain, we're open to new information and we're more likely to learn from our mistakes. Possibly most important, when we are uncertain, we are open to advice and input from other people.

When we are uncertain, we may ask ourselves, why? What is the source of this uncertainty? Is it because I don't know, or because it's not knowable? The first perspective is a personal attribution of uncertainty. That can make us feel deficient and put us on the path to strive toward more certainty, to remove the feeling of being unsure. But the other, more reasonable, perspective is that nobody knows. This is a universal attribution of uncertainty. Sure, I don't know, but neither do you nor does anyone else. That is: The knowledge I seek is unknowable with total certainty.

When we make a *personal attribution for our uncertainty*, essentially saying to ourselves, "I don't know but you do," we may pretend to know so we can save face and we feel stressed. When, instead, we make a *universal attribution for our uncertainty*, we realize that we're no different from anybody else no matter how certain they may seem to be, because certainty is an illusion. When we recognize this, it's easy to be confident and uncertain.

Uncertainty may be the key to health. By embracing it, we can leverage the uncertainty and find the advantage in the variability rather than avoiding it. A mindful body prospers from noticing change.

SYMPTOM VARIABILITY

Many older adults suffer memory lapses, which can lead them to worry that they will soon not be able to remember anything. Family members often share that belief and treat the older person as increasingly fragile and unaware. It's not uncommon to see people who need to get information about an elderly person ignore the elderly person and ask the person who is accompanying him or her for the information—instead of asking the elderly person for the information about himself or herself.

I was embarrassed to realize I made a similar assumption about my father in the last year of his life.

My father had been suffering from mild cognitive impairment. One day, when I was playing gin rummy with him, I presumed he couldn't remember the cards that had been thrown during the game. As I struggled with myself as to whether or not to let him win, he put down his cards and gleefully announced gin. I sheepishly realized my own mistake: Mild cognitive impairment may have stolen some memories from him, but of course there were things he could remember.

Years later, my graduate student Katherine Bercovitz and postdoc Karyn Gunnet-Shoval and I studied this more formally.[3] We asked adults aged sixty-five to eighty who were concerned about their memory to notice the fluctuations in their ability to remember things over the course of a week. In a text-message-based intervention, participants were asked to rate their memory twice per day, noticing how it differed from time to time and asking themselves why they might have been experiencing the fluctuations. As predicted, we found positive effects of the intervention, with those in the group who'd been asked to notice variation reporting significantly fewer memory lapses and more feelings of control over their memory after the intervention than before. On the other hand, we found that those who were asked to pay attention simply to their memory performance (but not the fluctuation) reported a lack of confidence in their ability to improve their memory.

We implemented a parallel intervention for chronic pain patients, texting them twice per day for one week to ask them to pay attention to the changes in their pain levels and asking them to make sense of the variability. We found that paying attention to the variability in the intensity of their pain resulted in positive changes including significant decreases in reports of pain interfering in their daily lives. The attention-to-variability intervention also resulted in a decreased likelihood that they would accept pain as a permanent fixture in their lives and an increased appreciation for communicating with their physician about their symptoms.

I conducted another pain study with my Israeli colleagues Noga Tsur and Ruth Defrin and members of my lab, but this time in Tsur and Defrin's lab in Israel.[4] If you've ever gotten a numbing shot in your mouth at the dentist's office, you may have noticed they put pressure on another part of your mouth when they give you the shot. It seems wholly unnecessary, but it works because when we have two sources of pain, they tend to balance each other out. In other words, for healthy people, the dentist putting pressure on your mouth means you'll feel less pain with the needle than otherwise. But for *some* people with chronic pain, that's unfortunately not true. Their pain does not diminish, and they feel the needle as painfully as if it were done alone. We wanted to know if an attention-to-variability treatment would result in less pain for them and lead them to feel more like a healthy person. We also tested the effects of a general mindfulness treatment that involved active noticing of non-pain-related visual images.

In this study, participants put their hand in very hot water after receiving training in attention to pain variability, mindful noticing, or a no-treatment control. The procedure was complicated, but the results were not. Both attention to variability and the general mindfulness treatment worked like a charm; the control group, however, continued to feel the pain.

In recent years our lab at Harvard has explored mind-body effects in diseases regarded as intractable. Lab members Francesco Pagnini, Deborah Phillips, Colin Bosma, Andrew Reece, and I collected correlational data on patients with ALS, a progressive nervous system disease that weakens muscles and breaks down nerve cells and which has no known medical cure.[5] We administered the Langer Mindfulness Scale to ALS patients and found a slower loss of function in those with higher mindfulness scores.

Once we knew that there was a correlational relationship between loss of function and mindfulness for people with ALS, we wanted to increase active noticing of the variability in their symptoms. Participants watched brief lectures about the main tenets of mindfulness: understanding uncertainty; the importance of noticing symptom variability; generating novelty; and recognizing that evaluations of good/bad are in our heads, not the external world. Then they engaged in exercises demonstrating each of these points.

One exercise involved manipulating a wheelchair. We wanted the ALS patients to focus on specifics. Among other things, we asked them to pay attention to how they gripped the wheel, what muscles they were using, and how that changed as they maneuvered from stopping to starting; where it is that they are gripping the wheel while it is at rest; and what part of their hand and which fingers they used.

The participants completed two mindfulness exercises, noticing minor changes daily for five weeks. We also had a control group that was given educational information about ALS and all the same measures we gave to the experimental group. It is not surprising that people who have ALS are often anxious and depressed, so we assessed anxiety and depression when we first started the study, and again after the intervention and at three- and six-months follow-up. We found that this intervention, which required a relatively short time commitment from patients, and was easy to do, was associated with improved psychological health for people with ALS: We saw a significant reduction of depression and anxiety in those who received the exercises compared to the control group. We are now conducting a follow-up to look at physical symptoms and overall well-being.

Members of my lab and I are also researching a good number of other chronic illnesses, including new and follow-up work on ALS, diabetes, Parkinson's disease, mild cognitive impairment, multiple sclerosis, stroke, and depression. In each study, we teach the patient—and/or their caregiver where possible or appropriate—to attend to symptom variability to adopt a mindful approach to controlling the effects of the specific disorder. We have preliminary results so far from research on MS,[6] stroke,[7] and Parkinson's disease that are very promising.

When it comes to disabilities, people have alternative abilities and can even do some of what they have come to believe their disability denies them. For instance, people with one leg may think they can't play football and thus are different from the rest of us until they see that many of us with two legs also can't play football. Indeed, one approach to reducing outgroup bias may be to increase in-group discrimination. Once we see that none of us is us, "they" don't look so different.

Body parts have numerous functions. To say something doesn't work is much too global. Too often we define ourselves by what is lacking rather than what is there. The more mindful a person is, the more open and aware of change they will be and, as a result, the more resilient. The helpless person sees all situations as the same. The mindful person notices the differences and thus becomes more resilient. A simple example: Even if we've been certified as disabled and have the blue parking permit to prove it, sometimes we don't need to park in the handicapped space.

Because mind and body are taken as one, mind-body unity predicts that what is true for our physical health is also true for our mental health. Attention to variability treatments, for example, also may be effective for people whose health issue is clinical depression. One of the stable beliefs held by people who are depressed is that their condition is not going to improve. There is no light at the end of the tunnel. But no one's depression is exactly the same from moment to moment nor from day to day. Noticing small improvements in how we feel may provide insights into our depression just as with physical symptoms. Attention-to-variability treatments may be useful for mental illnesses that the medical world may assume are intractable. With serious illnesses like schizophrenia, for example, rather than expecting the person suffering from symptoms to attend to their variability, perhaps the clinician can do the monitoring.

We can apply attention to variability not only to chronic disease but also to behaviors like wanting to smoke less or drink less or even eat less. Heavy drinkers and chain-smokers and binge eaters may think they always want a drink, a cigarette, or a candy bar. As discussed above, if we kept a diary in which we regularly recorded whether we wanted the substance or not and whether we did or didn't actually have it, we'd come to see that despite what we thought, in reality we don't always want it. More important, we'd come to see that we are in charge—not the alcohol, cigarette, or piece of cake.

HEALING IS A MATTER OF OPPORTUNITY

I remember how helpless I felt a good deal of the time I spent with my mother when she was in the hospital. If I had been encouraged to help her by noticing her changing symptoms and helping her to notice them as well, I probably would have felt better. Across a good number of our studies, no matter what ailment we're examining, we've found that when we increase mindfulness in general, attend to variations in symptoms, and include caregivers in the process, people show meaningful improvement. Much of the data I've reported over the years has also made clear that not only are these mindful approaches good for health and disease, they actually feel good.

Imagine if medical staff in a nursing home or hospital were to make note every day of how each resident is different from the day before. To do this, they would have to pay a different kind of attention to the resident. Some staff might feel that adding noticing differences to their list of responsibilities would make their job harder, but I think instead, it would make their jobs more interesting. Caregiver burnout is real, and turnover in hospital and nursing home staff is a problem. By increasing mindfulness in the medical staff, some of the monotony of caretaking responsibilities and the pressure and stress that results would diminish. Further, by noticing the physical changes in their patients, caregivers may become more attentive to their patients' emotional states. If caregivers did this mindful noticing, I think it would result in patients' feeling seen, and many would come to savor their relationships with the medical staff. Decades of research have shown that mindfulness increases health. Ironically, better, more nuanced attention to hospital patients and nursing home residents should—by this logic—improve the health of the staff as well.

Dr. Rita Charon's book *Narrative Medicine* introduced me to a movement in medicine that relates closely to a mind-body approach.[8] By listening to the patient's story, physicians come to see how unique each person is. Perceiving this singularity is one of the hallmarks of mindfulness. By actively noticing unique attributes in their patients, physicians can stay attentive and engaged. When they see their doctors are mindfully attentive, people feel seen, stress subsides, and healing unfolds. Dr. Charon writes, "Sometimes, it is as if doctor and patient were alien planets, aware of one another's trajectories only by traces of stray light and strange matter." Diagnosing patients' physical symptoms, without exploring what they mean to the patients, misses many opportunities to treat them. Listening expands the possibility of treatment. For example, an eighty-nine-year-old patient of Dr. Charon's had many pains unexplained by her tests and diagnoses. It was not until Dr. Charon found out that she had been raped as a young child and never told anyone about it that the woman opened up, and as a result, her pain diminished, and her health was restored.

When we have a medical disorder, there is a tendency to understand every ache and pain as arising from the condition. Surely, for at least some of our physical problems, there are alternative explanations. When health professionals mindlessly assume every symptom is part of the disease they've diagnosed or are treating, they give up the possibility to potentially influence the course of a patient's illness. Diagnoses, while useful, direct attention to only a fraction of lived experience; context influences our physical responses.

We think in the general but act in the specific. We want to lose weight in the abstract but eat the chocolate bar in front of our face. Sometimes, broad generalizations blind us to specific counterexamples. When we feel depressed, we may be too depressed to notice the specific times when we are less depressed, or not depressed at all.

Attention to variability can help solve this problem. When we are paying attention to variability, we may more quickly notice new symptoms. Attention to variability should lead people to notice how they can influence their conditions and pinpoint the problem.

Of course, the first step to an attention-to-variability solution is to recognize that improvement may be possible. As I've repeatedly argued, we can never know that we can't improve. All science can tell us is that we can improve or that the verdict is still out. When we believe that, like Humpty-Dumpty, once we fall apart and experience diminished performance, and all of the king's horses and all of the king's men can't put us back together again, we feel helpless. Perhaps for many of us all we really need is to be told that improvement is possible and then we can begin our own journey to figure out how to do it. If so, we'd come on our own to attend to variability. We expect improvement and then attend to signs of the medication/treatment/expectation working. Doing so we come to recognize the circumstances when it does work and when it doesn't, and we can use that information to help us heal. This may also explain how placebos work. Once we take a placebo we look for improvement.

Sometimes it's not easy to notice the ways our pain, for example, changes. Nevertheless, to my mind it is well worth the time figuring it out. One can easily see how these truths can be applied to diagnosing and treating disease in the medical world.

Noticing variability speaks to how diseases may be better understood and studied as conditions in flux rather than static; how diagnoses that ignore moment-to-moment changes are probably better as starting points to gather more data rather than final conclusions; how caregivers might improve their care by attending to subtle differences in those to whom they are giving care; and—most relevant here—how people may learn a different way to experience their medical conditions.

When taken together, all of this work on attention to variability show us that the simple act of noticing change may have enormous consequences for our health. Indeed it may not be the strongest of the species that survive, but rather those most responsive to change.

Four things happen when we notice the variability of our symptoms. First, we see that despite what we may have thought, we don't have the symptom all the time and to the same degree, and that itself should make us feel better. Second, noticing change is mindful, and decades of our research have shown that mindfulness itself is good for our health. Third, we're more likely to find a solution to our problem if we search for it than if we remain helpless and mindlessly presume there is no relief available. And fourth, we start to feel more in control of our lives.

We develop an awareness of variability by tracking changes across time and context. Noticing changes in different parts of our bodies—our sensations, emotions, thoughts, and environments—is empowering as well. Every person differs from the mean in different ways. Science essentially averages these differences away and treats them like noise. But this "noise" may be hiding the key to our health. Moreover, rather than focus on the normative response, these outliers may be extremely important. It's important to ask, why does this person *not* conform to the norm?

The future will be different from the past. What to do with all this uncertainty? Notice what is happening now.

CHAPTER 9

Mindful Contagion

Pure truth cannot be assimilated by the crowd.
It must be communicated by contagion.
—Henri-Frédéric Amiel

We've all had the experience of being drawn to some people without a clear idea of why. They seem to have a special je ne sais quoi that's unusually charming and appealing. Similarly, we've all had the experience of being turned off by someone who seemed more robot than flesh-and-blood human. Reflecting on this made me think that we may be unwittingly responding to how mindful or mindless the other person may be. Since I have a clear preference to be with people who are mindful, it occurred to me that maybe it is possible to become more mindful oneself simply by being in the presence of a mindful person.

But before I could examine the extent to which mindfulness might be contagious, I wanted to know if most people are, in fact, drawn to people who are mindful. I discussed this idea many years ago with my colleague John Sviokla, when I spent a semester at Harvard Business School. We decided to test it with a group of magazine salesmen whom we randomly assigned to one of two groups.[1] Salesmen in the first group were asked to approach each new customer in exactly the same way and to use exactly the same sales pitch with each one of their potential new customers. The salesmen in the second group were told to vary their pitch and to adopt a more mindful approach. We asked them to make each sales pitch new in subtle ways each time they approached a new customer.

Customers who received the mindful sales pitches described those salesmen as charismatic. These customers were also more likely to purchase magazines than those who had listened to the mindless sales pitches. This work provided initial evidence that mindfulness is readily perceived by others and can in turn shape their behavior.

I began to wonder whether animals perceive mindfulness as they interacted with people. I first studied this by bringing my dogs to the lab and asking each lab member one at a time to be mindless (repeating overlearned thoughts like the nursery rhyme "Mary had a little lamb") or be mindful (thinking novel thoughts like "What if Mary brought a fox instead of a lamb to school with her?"). I noted whose company the dogs sought, and it seemed to work—the dogs were more attracted to the mindful person. But these were my dogs, and I understood that other factors might have been at play: If the dogs approached someone because they sensed the person, in some way, was like me—the person who fed them and gave them treats—it might have nothing to do with mindfulness per se.

Undeterred, I moved the experiment to a kennel that

boarded dogs while their owners were away; the staff was game to help me test dogs for awareness of human mindfulness. To start, I divided the staff into two groups. One group was trained to think novel thoughts about nursery rhymes when they were with the dogs, while the other was asked to just keep repeating the same rhyme to themselves. Did it make a difference as to which person a dog preferred? It seemed to, but unfortunately the chaos of the kennel—the barking, the constant activity—made it impossible to draw any firm conclusions. It occurred to me that I was more interested in whether people noticed mindfulness in other people than in dogs having this awareness. So, the next step was to test the idea with children who might be better behaved than the dogs. At least the incessant barking would be gone.

It was the end of the school year, so we decided to run the study at a boys' summer camp.[2] We randomly assigned the campers to one of two groups and planned to have our researcher interview the boys in each group posing as coaches visiting from another camp. The first group of interviewers was instructed to be mindful by carefully noticing changes in a child—both verbal and nonverbal—over the course of the interview. The second group of interviewers was directed to be mindless, only pretending to be interested in what a camper had to say. In both cases the interviewers were told the interviews should be positive. After the interviews, campers were given a test that measured their self-esteem and asked about their camp experience. When running experiments in which participants are randomly assigned to a group, it is assumed that the boys in the two groups were equivalent on all measures of concern at the start. But after the experiment, the campers were quite different. The children who interacted with a mindless adult had significantly lower self-esteem scores and an expressed dislike of both the camp and the interviewer than campers interacting with a mindful adult. Interacting with a mindful adult had a positive effect on the campers. Not only did they have higher self-esteem and like the camp more, they were happier and more likely to think the interviewer liked them.

CATCHING MINDFULNESS

As I noted above, we have all experienced interacting with people who appear to be more "magnetic" than others: They seem to have a presence that we find appealing. Is mindfulness behind this effect? We first played with the idea of mindful contagion in pilot work in our lab. A participant entered the room and was seated almost shoulder to shoulder next to another student, who was actually a research assistant and a member of our team who had been instructed, in advance, to be mindful by quietly noticing new things in the room. In half of the cases, however, the experimenter was instructed to be mindless by focusing on counting to one hundred. After a minute or two, the participant was given an index card that had a slightly flawed version of a familiar phrase printed on it. Instead of "Mary had a little lamb" it read "Mary had a a little lamb." After reading it, they gave the card back, and were asked to then repeat what they had read. Virtually everyone repeated Mary had a little lamb—without the double word. We asked how many words were on the card and they all said "five." But when in close proximity to someone mindful, people were more likely to notice the double letter. This test of noticing is a simple but effective measure of mindfulness. While everyone ordinarily misses the slight change in the familiar phrase, decades ago when we gave the index card to people who'd just finished meditating, they all read the card correctly.

Right before the Covid pandemic, Dr. Daoning Zhang from the Beijing University of Chinese Medicine was visiting my lab. She thought the contagion research fit well with the Chinese concept of chi and wanted to replicate it once she returned to China. The Chinese were interested in seeing if mindful contagion could be measured by high-frequency terahertz brain waves. Not knowing anything about brain waves, my lab manager, Kris Nichols, and I were more interested in learning if we could replicate the mindful noticing finding we got earlier.

As they were measuring the brain activity of participants, Dr. Zhang's research assistants were instructed to look at the participants' hands and either mindfully notice subtle details—were the hands wrinkled, calloused, or red in some spots?—or simply mindlessly focus on them. Immediately following the process, each participant was given an index card and asked to read aloud the Chinese proverb that was printed on it. Again, every card had a misprint; a repeated word in the proverb.

It turned out that the research assistants' mindfulness was indeed contagious. As Dr. Zhang reported to me, 24 out of 25 participants who were in the presence of an assistant who was paying mindful attention to their hands saw the repeated word, and these participants also showed an overall increase in brain wave activity. For those who were in the mindless group, only 11 out of 70 participants saw the error.

It might seem like a leap of logic that one person's attention to someone else's hands, of all things, leads to greater awareness. But this idea of mindful contagion no longer seems bizarre to me. And if true, is there a way to reap its benefits beyond just seeing an overlooked printed word?

SENSITIVITY TO MINDFULNESS

If mindful contagion is real, it isn't necessarily the case that we are all equally affected by exposure to it. It is likely that some of us are more susceptible to the differences between mindfulness and mindlessness in others, and mindful contagion might have clinical implications.

To test if this is the case, members of my lab and I looked at whether people who drink to numb themselves do so in whole or in part because they are hypersensitive to interpersonal cues that indicate whether another person is mindless or not. It is uncomfortable to be around people who are mindless. Perhaps a drink is one way for sensitive adults to lessen the effect.

My lab members John Allman, Kris Nichols, and I first tested this indirectly. Forty self-reported problem drinkers were recruited at open Alcoholics Anonymous meetings in Cambridge, Massachusetts. Open meetings are available to anyone interested in the AA program of recovery from problem drinking. The meeting secretary announced that our study would take place after the meeting and that participation was both completely voluntary and confidential. Along with the volunteers from the AA meeting, an additional forty participants with no reported history of alcohol misuse were used as a comparison group.

Each of the eighty participants was asked to join our study on "person perception" and have a short conversation with one of our research assistants. The research assistants were instructed to ask the volunteers a series of questions—such as "Did you have a good day or a bad day today?" and "What are the pros and cons of trying to break a bad habit in a group of peers?"

Half of the research assistants were instructed to be mindful when they were asking these questions and to pay attention to individual characteristics of the participant (such as eye color, likely socioeconomic status, appearance, and behavior). They were told "Try to keep in mind that all participants are different and that by observing differences among different participants, you can learn important information about a person's perspective."

The second half of the research assistants were assigned to be mindless and to just pretend that they were interested in the participants' answers to the questions. These research assistants were told "Participants are all pretty much the same, but please pretend that you are interested in the answers from all of them." They didn't say anything different from the mindful interviewers. They simply were less engaged in the conversation.

After five minutes, regardless of the number of questions completed, the research assistants ended the conversation. But before they did so, they all asked one last question: Would the participant like to continue to be a participant in our study?

Our hypothesis was that those interviewed by someone mindless would be less likely to agree to be in the study, and we were right. It turns out that other people's mindlessness probably affects all of us, but some more than others: Fewer people from the AA group than the nondrinker group were inclined to stick with the study if they had been interviewed by a mindless assistant not really interested in their answers. This was the first indication that heavy drinkers might be more sensitive to how mindless the people around them may be. It's not clear what links drinking to this sensitivity, whether it is genetic or learned, but my concern was with the potential flip side of this sensitivity: Are drinkers sensitive to other people's mindlessness?

John, Kris, and I continued this line of inquiry. We set out to determine whether people interacting with a mindless experimenter were more inclined to drink.

This time we recruited sixty adults from the Harvard community and greater Boston area. We told the participants that the study was measuring the effects of emotion on wine taste. We ask them to refrain from drinking anything for an hour before the experiment.

Next, we recruited a cohort of people to pose as our experimenters. These people were unaware of our hypothesis, and we randomly assigned them to either the mindful or mindless condition. We gave the mindful experimenters detailed instructions on how to view the participants as individuals, to notice things about them such as their clothes, their hair, how tall they were, and, most important, how they changed over the course of their participation. Mindless experimenters were instructed to smile, be nice to participants, and follow the script.

Before proceeding with the study, we measured the participant in two ways: We assessed their mindfulness using the Langer Mindfulness Scale and asked them to complete the World Health Organization's Alcohol Use Disorder Identification Test, to help in the self-assessment of alcohol consumption. Once those questionnaires were completed, participants were interviewed, by either a mindful or mindless interviewer. The interview consisted of general questions about mood and attitude toward the wine-tasting task. The script was similar to the AA study described above.

When the interview was done, we told the participants that they would be taking part in a wine-tasting experiment. The experimenter indicated that they could drink as much wine as they wanted, and then asked them to complete a taste survey. While the amount of wine consumed was what we were interested in, to participants it seemed like a wine-tasting study: We asked participants to rank the wine they drank on a scale of 1 to 10 and come up with an estimated price of a bottle of the wine. We also asked them to provide a list of any flavors or tastes they had noticed.

Our hypothesis was confirmed. Those participants who were in the presence of a mindful experimenter drank half as much alcohol. Those in the presence of the mindless experimenter drank four ounces versus only two ounces for those in the presence of the mindful experimenter. In this context where participants are typically concerned with how they may be evaluated, this difference is meaningful.

These results were not gathered to show that drinking itself is any more or less a mindful activity than abstaining, but simply that, to the extent that one of the features of excessive use of alcohol is as a way to "escape" reality, the more mindful we are, the less we feel a need to escape. Thus, the results suggest mindfulness is contagious—interacting with someone mindful increases our own mindfulness.

I've since continued to explore mindful contagion in a study of children with autism spectrum disorders. I wanted to know if autistic children reacted in the same way that the heavy drinkers did and were also more sensitive to other people's mindlessness or mindfulness. Put another way: Since most people are mindless most of the time, and mindlessness is interpersonally uncomfortable, can sensitivity to mindlessness explain some of the interpersonal challenges of people with autism? I wasn't setting out to study whether autism creates this sensitivity or whether this sensitivity is the result of the confluence of many factors that result from the condition. My interest was simply in seeing if there is a relationship between sensitivity to mindlessness/mindfulness and being on the spectrum.

Together with my postdocs Francesco Pagnini and Deborah Phillips and a group of Italian researchers, we tested this in an Italian community. Autistic children interacted with mindless or mindful adults, and their behavior was noted. We enlisted eight children who were similar in their level of functioning on the autism spectrum and six adult assistants to participate in the study. We assigned the pairings randomly— some children would interact with a mindful adult and others would be working with a less mindful one. During the thirty-minute sessions, we gave each child three games to play with the adult experimenter. We videotaped the sessions, and independent raters subsequently coded the videos for both verbal and nonverbal interactive behaviors.

The adults in the low-mindful condition were instructed to pretend to be interested in what the child was doing and to be positive in all that they said to the child. We provided no other instructions about how they should behave. The adults in the high-mindful condition received the same instructions with the additional instruction to focus on the variability of the child's behavior and the emergence of novel elements in their emotional expression. That is, we asked them to observe how the child's body language, voice inflection, and general state of being changed over the course of the interview and to consider what varied or remained the same as they played the games. We suggested that they study the child to understand their internal state, just as they might glean hints about a painter's internal state by studying a painting.

When these children interacted with the mindful adults, they showed a greater number of "fun behaviors." They interacted more with the experimenters and showed fewer avoidance behaviors. They showed an increase in collaborative behaviors and a decrease in stereotyped behaviors. The mindfulness of the adults appeared to make the children more mindful (implying contagion) and led to their more engaged interaction.

In the past, scientists studying autism have been quick to say that autistic children have trouble "reading" the emotional nonverbal behavior of adults. Most of the research concerned the information we get from other people's eyes. For example, our pupils are dilated when we are attracted to someone. More recently, however, research has found that children on the spectrum were underestimated. They are actually quite skilled at reading body language when full-body posture is taken into account. Our work in Italy suggests that these children are perhaps skilled at reading our states of mind as well.

I also think it's worth questioning whether part of the problem many adults have in connecting with children on the autism spectrum lies with the adults and not the children. These adults may have difficulty "reading" the cues that autistic children display, or be unmotivated to try to do so because of their biases. If adults were more mindful, they would be more sensitive to those cues and would probably interact better with the children.

MINDFUL CONTAGION AND HEALTH

As more than forty years of research has shown, mindfulness is good for our health. The research on mindful contagion suggests that one person's mindfulness may increase another person's mindfulness. Thus, I think it may be the case that the people around us with whom we interact may actually be having a positive effect on our health.

To wit: In a study conducted in Switzerland, my postdoc Chiara Haller and I examined 176 patients suffering from severe traumatic brain injury and the relatives who were the primary caregivers.[3] We found a correlation between the mindfulness of the caregiver and the functioning of the patient. One explanation may be that mindful caregivers are likely to attend to the variability in symptoms and responses of those for whom they are caring. I suspect that mindful contagion may also play a part. A caregiver's mindfulness may increase the mindfulness of those for whom they are caring.

These studies also have a bearing on the ill health that too often results for caregivers who care for people with chronic illnesses or for elderly people with memory problems. I believe illness among caregivers results from the stress of a mindless, fixed view that symptoms will only get worse. Caught up in a negative mindset, they give and give until they feel empty. But when caregivers start to notice small changes in the symptoms of the people for whom they are caring, several things happen. They become more mindful themselves, which as we saw earlier is good for their own health. And when caregivers are more engaged and optimistic, their jobs seem a bit easier, and burnout becomes less likely.

This work also has implications for people with mild cognitive impairment. Imagine that you're caring for someone who suffers from severe memory loss. He asks you a question, you answer it, and then moments later he asks it again. And again, you answer. With each passing exchange, your frustration may be growing. It's hard to remember that the forgetting isn't willful. But when people recognize that it is unlikely that their loved one is forgetting everything, opportunity presents itself. Why is one thing being forgotten and not another? Exploring the answer is good for both participants.

This way of thinking is relevant for other disorders as well. Consider dyslexia. If the person with dyslexia recognized that letters or words aren't always transposed, trying to figure out which ones are, and why, could turn frustration into the engaging task of solving a puzzle. Why is this word a problem in this context but not in others? A negative mindset leads us to focus only on the negative. Indeed, often much of what's on the page is read correctly. If we realized the likely infrequency of errors, we'd be less inclined to blame ourselves or others for them. It feels better to get most of it right rather than noticing only when something goes wrong. What this really amounts to is a move from global thinking (everything, always) to specific instances (some words, sometimes). This makes solutions easier to see.

OUR SENSES

The blind have a keener and more nuanced sense of hearing than those of us who have their sight intact. And for the deaf, sight becomes more important and thus enhanced. Indeed, they even have heightened peripheral vision. It seems to me, rather than use norms to assess what we can and cannot do, it would be better to investigate those who are superior on a particular dimension and see if we can learn from them.

The point here is, if someone else can do it, the rest of us could as well, albeit even if more slowly. Rather than see people like Einstein and Mozart—or the blind and the deaf—as outliers, we should understand that they reveal more of what is possible than impossible. One may ask why, as we age, doesn't our hearing improve as our vision worsens? I would answer that it is because we have strong negative mindsets about aging. These mindsets convince us that as we get older, our senses must deteriorate. But there aren't the same negative mindsets that tell the deaf they cannot sharpen their vision or the blind that they cannot develop their hearing.

Among the most debilitating mindsets is the expectation that our memory must worsen as we age. But it does not worsen for everyone and it does not always get worse for those who live without that mindset. This is what Yale psychologist Becca Levy and I found when Becca was my graduate student at Harvard.[4] We conducted research with participants who we thought had this age bias along with those who did not assume memory worsens with age. Our hypothesis was that the *belief* that memory problems increase with age leads to memory problems.

We included old and young Chinese participants, since the Chinese typically have more respect for elders than Americans do, and so they are less likely to believe that memory must worsen over time. We also believed that people who are deaf are unlikely to buy into the negative aging mindset since they have enough to deal with in a world controlled by those who can hear, and so we included young and old people who are deaf in the study.

We found that among the American participants with intact hearing, the young outperformed the old on memory tests, reflecting what most Americans take as a necessary consequence of aging. This was not true, however, for the deaf and Chinese populations. In these cases, the older subjects' ability to remember was just as strong as the young.

We have solid evidence that dogs can be taught to smell whether an individual has cancer. Heather Junqueira and her colleagues taught four beagles to discriminate between blood samples from healthy people and lung cancer patients.[5] One of the dogs apparently couldn't have cared less about the importance of the research, but the other three correctly identified the lung cancer patients 97 percent of the time. Can we learn to improve our ability to smell to a similar degree? If we could, we might detect cancer in ourselves or others much sooner and thereby save lives. There are those who will say the biology of the pigeon, dog, ant, or crocodile gives them acute senses that are impossible for us to acquire. To this I say, "Maybe" but also "Maybe not." If a person can lift 150 pounds, it doesn't mean they need all of their muscle power to lift 50 pounds. Just because dogs have five times the number of olfactory receptors in their noses as humans do, it doesn't mean that their 300 million receptors are necessary to sniff out cancer. Dogs are said to have neophilia, that is, they are attracted to new scents, while people tend to be attracted to familiar scents. But that doesn't mean we can't learn to be mindful and notice unfamiliar odors.

Undaunted by the naysayers, members of my lab and I considered testing whether we could improve people's sense of smell and, if so, could they successfully smell whether someone had cancer? This hypothesis may not be quite as extreme as it first appears to be. After designing our study, I came upon an article about a person named Joy Milne, who had the ability to smell Parkinson's disease.[6] In a test, she was able to accurately identify T-shirts belonging to people both with and without Parkinson's. She made only one "error": She identified a person as having Parkinson's who, at the time, was thought not to have Parkinson's. And then, a few months later, he was diagnosed with it. Clearly, cancer and Parkinson's are different diseases, but the idea of a human being able to smell disease is quite possible.

We've just begun looking into this, so we'll have to wait some time for the results to see if people can be taught to improve their sense of smell enough to detect diseases. Our intention is to ask people who have cancer and their spouses (as control participants) to sleep in a T-shirt that we will provide to them. The next morning, they will put their shirts in separate ziplock bags and return them to us. We will then test if the participants' sense of smell can be enhanced through exercises such that they are able to identify beyond chance the shirts worn by those who have cancer. But even if the training fails, it does not mean the broader hypothesis is wrong. It could be that more or different training is necessary.

To live in a world of endless possibilities means that so-called challenges will be commonplace because we are trying things that have never been done before, either by us or by society. But to do that which is uncommon, or what the world doesn't actively promote, or for which there are unwritten rules against moving forward, is not as challenging as it might at first seem.

The word "challenge" for many conjures up suffering and the real possibility of failure. But we need to turn it around and ask ourselves what success feels like the moment after we catch our breath. We're left to ask ourselves, "Now what?" I'm fond of using the challenging game of golf as an example. If we were finally getting a hole in one every time we swung the golf club, the game would no longer be any fun. We can either do a task imperfectly mindfully or perfectly mindlessly. When we behave mindlessly, the experience is empty. Failure then needs to be understood as incomplete success; unless you give up, there is no such thing as failure.

Many years ago, a news program was doing a segment on my first nursing home study. I suggested they open the segment with a person asking how much the audience would like a life with no challenges, one in which everything was done for us. And then pan to a nursing home. They didn't use my suggestion. I was arguing even then for making life in a nursing home more challenging rather than accepting an environment that promotes mindlessness.

Several years ago, Peso, our rescue dog, stole food we had put out in the living room for guests. He's typically well-behaved and gentle, but that night, he behaved like, well, a dog. We quickly scolded him, and my partner decided Peso needed to go to obedience school.

If you asked us whether we expect perfection from Peso, we'd be quick to answer, "Of course not." Perhaps a 90 percent success rate, but never perfection. On the other hand, like everyone else, we rarely consider an instance of misbehavior as part of the 10 percent. Instead, we mindlessly view it as failure.

It's the same way we tend to treat older adults. If your parent or grandparent fumbles with the key when trying to open a locked door, we may take the keys and open it ourselves, acting as though we've never struggled with a lock. If he or she falls, we not only rush to help—which may be a good thing—but we take note to make sure it never happens again—which may be a bad thing. And if she or he forgets something we deem worth remembering, we start looking for signs of dementia and take each petty instance of forgetting thereafter as evidence.

If we confined our pets to a cage or if we induced a semi-comatose state in older adults, we could make sure misdeeds didn't occur. There would be no failure, falling, nor forgetfulness. Whether beast or beauty, to be alive is to be imperfect, welcoming challenges and uncertainty, and that should be perfectly fine at every age.

Remember when we were young and reaching the elevator button was challenging? Now that we're grown up and taller, how often does hitting the button result in glee? We enjoyed tic-tac-toe until we learned how to win or tie every time. We are unlikely to deem it fun to work on a crossword puzzle we successfully completed yesterday if we remember all or most of the answers. If we were able to score a hole in one in golf with every swing, there'd be no game to play. If we really wanted to always win any particular game, we could play against children. In practice, we prefer a challenge to guaranteed success. It's the struggle that's fun.

Facing a challenge can feel overwhelming, but we can deal with it by taking one small step after another. It is not just from big acorns that mighty oaks grow. In almost all my research, we have shown that small changes can have enormous impact. In my first study with elderly adults, we found that simply giving nursing home residents small, mundane choices resulted in longer lives.[7]

In another early study, we made remembering matter in a reasonably innocuous way by asking nursing home residents to remember things like nurses' names and receive tokens for success.[8] The task increased in difficulty every week. The subjects' memories improved, even though the prevailing myth was that memory only worsens over time. In study after study conducted over the past forty-some years, we've found that with only subtle shifts in our thinking and expectations, we can begin to change the ingrained behaviors that sap health, competence, optimism, and vitality from our lives.

As more people come to appreciate and exploit the power of uncertainty, a mindful utopia may be closer than many think. Once we recognize that it is simply decisions from the past that are limiting us, there is little stopping us from redesigning the world to better fit our current needs rather than using yesterday to determine today and tomorrow. When we do this, that which was previously taken as impossible may yield to a new view of the unimpossible. Why not?

SOMETHING IN THE AIR

Are there certain places where large numbers of people gather that are prone to elicit mindfulness? Many of us have experienced this effect informally, whether in beautifully landscaped green spaces, concert halls listening to great music, or holy places. In each of these contexts we slow down and take in the beauty or grandeur before us. Is there something about the place that leads us to be more mindful, or is it just our expectation that there is something important to notice and so we do?

It's easy to test whether and in what contexts people have had this experience; all we need to do is ask them. If it's something about the place, testing how to explain these experiences is a different matter. Our current understanding of science does not offer satisfactory mechanisms for explaining sensations that might linger in a physical environment. But, nevertheless, it may still be an important, albeit unusual, area of study.

When Clayton McClintock was a Harvard student and a member of my lab, we took a bold step in this direction with a study we later called "Something in the Air." We were essentially interested in seeing whether participants who were given tasks in a room in which meditators had just finished meditating would outperform those who took the same tests in a room that was not previously occupied. Was there something in the air that would affect their performance? The experiment took place in a small classroom that could seat twelve people comfortably around a conference table. There were three groups of participants, all of whom took simple cognitive tests before the experiment began. In the experimental condition, participants were guided into an empty room where the meditators had just meditated together, practicing an insight-style meditation, where one becomes aware of thoughts and sensations arising within one's awareness without focusing on these thoughts and sensations. After meditating for approximately forty-five minutes, they received a signal from a researcher and quietly and inconspicuously left the classroom and building. The desks, chairs, and other furniture weren't disturbed in any way and the room temperature was held constant.

In one of the two comparison groups, instead of meditators a group of people sat in the room and watched a video that had been designed to elicit stressful emotions. It included footage from a tsunami and a kidney operation, as well as graphic highway safety footage. After approximately forty-five minutes, they too received a signal from a researcher to exit quietly and carefully from the classroom and building. The desks, chairs, and other furniture again remained in the same arrangement as before arrival.

In the last comparison group, the room was left unoccupied for forty-five minutes before the research participants arrived.

While the meditators were meditating, or the comparison group was watching the film, sixty-eight participants were gathered in smaller groups at another part of the campus and were asked to complete a questionnaire. The researchers informed the participants that they would be visiting another room in the building, but they gave no description of the room. Before walking to the new room, the participants were told to remain quiet on the way and to pay attention to their impression of the room when they arrived there. The researchers then led groups of eight to twelve participants down the hall and into the classroom. Neither the participants nor the researchers with them were aware of whether the room had been previously occupied.

As soon as the participants took their seats, a researcher asked them to answer two questions using an eleven-point scale: "How appealing does this room feel?" (0 = Very Unappealing, 10 = Very Appealing) and "How enlivening does this room feel?" (0 = Very Unenlivening, 10 = Very Enlivening). We also measured reaction time using an application on a tablet in which participants tapped circles as soon as they noticed they lit up on the tablet screen. After ten taps, the program recorded how much time had elapsed, measuring how quickly participants noticed when the circle lit up to the nearest hundred-thousandth of a second.

The participants who came into the room after individuals had either watched the video or meditated reported that the room felt more enlivening and appealing than the people who entered the room that no one had previously been in. This supports the idea that there was something in the air in the rooms where people had recently been. If not, the three groups would have experienced the room in the same way.

More important, however, there were significant differences in the reaction times in the tapping exercise. Testing reaction time is perhaps the clearest measure of mindfulness. Noticing differences is the essence of mindfulness as we study it. The more mindful you are, the faster you notice differences and the quicker your reaction time will be. Those who occupied a room where meditators had just finished meditating had faster reaction times to the tablet screen color change than those who occupied a room where people had seen a video and those who were in a room that hadn't been occupied by anyone. The latter two groups were not meaningfully different.

These mysterious results suggest that somehow our mindfulness leaves a residue in the air and as such may affect the mindfulness of others. Without doing some follow-up investigations, these results should be understood as suggestive. It does seem, though, that in these situations "there is something in the air" that advanced technology may eventually reveal, just as in the past, predicting the gender of a fetus was seen as an intuition. Now with ultrasound, gender is apparent. A mother's intuition could have been a physical feeling. I believe that every internal action is accompanied by an external signifier—be it odor, perspiration, or energy emitted.

An incomplete explanation does not mean something does not reliably happen. The Something in the Air study suggests a cause and effect, even if we are not at the point of being able to describe or understand it. We are not sure how placebos work, yet we accept their power. I am neither a believer nor disbeliever in the existence of paranormal phenomena. The fact that I can't explain something does not incline me to disbelieve. I know I turn on my television and someone in New York appears in my house. I Zoom with my students and colleagues, and they appear on my computer. I don't really understand these events either, yet I accept them.

Ordinary explanations for common events also feel lacking. I eat because I am hungry. What does it really mean to understand, examine, and give names to internal processes? In general, we define things by changing the level of analysis. We either go down a level of analysis as in neuroscience explanations or we go up a level of explanation as sociological or philosophical understandings of behavior. But I'm not convinced that by doing so we're really any closer to understanding. No explanation is ever fully complete.

Remaining aware of the power of known unknowns may keep us open to the possibility of unknown unknowns. Seeing unusual phenomena as indeterminate rather than "impossible" allows today's impossible to become tomorrow's "but of course." There isn't a cost to staying open to possibility. But dismissing strange experiences because we can't explain them may only result in missed opportunities.

CHAPTER 10

Why Not?

Physiology will have nothing to do with them. Orthodox psychology turns its back upon them. Medicine sweeps them out; or, at most, when in an anecdotal vein, records a few of them as "effects of the imagination." . . . No matter where you open its pages, you find things recorded under the name of divinations, inspirations, demoniacal possessions, apparitions, trances, ecstasies, miraculous healings and productions of disease, and occult powers possessed by peculiar individuals over persons and things in their neighborhood.

—WILLIAM JAMES

William James, the father of American psychology and the namesake of the building in which I've spent most of my career, believed that science had failed us all by abandoning unusual phenomena.[1] He saw the tendency of scientists to prejudge what is possible or impossible as an error, and throughout his life tried to keep an open mind to all sorts of possibilities. I'm in his camp. I believe that the key to effective change lies in our recognizing that certainty imprisons free will.

Much has been written about blind obedience to authority, typically as it concerns institutional authority and not the more mundane instances where it doesn't even occur to us to question a rule or the apparent legitimacy of the "ruler." Imagine applying to college and being required to write an essay about your hero. The problem is you don't have a hero or can't name just one. What do you do? My guess is that most people will make something up or make a choice. Perhaps the choice would be Eleanor Roosevelt, Mother Teresa, or Abraham Lincoln. The better essay might be one that considers why we don't have a hero in the first place or one that considers an inability to name just one, but rarely do these alternatives even come to mind; most students just want to respond to the requirement.

Similarly, we are taught who is worthy of our esteem and often blindly accept the given criteria rather than explore what is meaningful to us personally. We tend to accept the premises implicit in questions. In that sense, all questions are "loaded" questions—especially when these are interview or application questions where we are hoping to join an exclusive community, or in other situations where there is a perceived power disparity. Consider the power disparity in a hospital.

What happens when a doctor asks a nurse to do something the nurse thinks is a mistake? It's hard to question the higher-status person. Moreover, we are obedient so often that frequently it doesn't even occur to us to consider the question. When we're given a prescription for a drug and have a mild negative reaction to it, do we feel comfortable telling the doctor we should have been given something else? Or do we continue following the doctor's orders to take it twice a day with food? We're told by a doctor that our broken leg will take six to eight weeks to heal. Does it even occur to us to try to get better in half the time?

What would happen if instead of being given an expectation for average healing time we were told the quickest known time someone took to heal? Would we heal faster? I believe we would. When I smashed my ankle, luckily I forgot that I was told that I would always walk with a limp. Whether I end up hitting the ball on the tennis court or miss it, there is no evidence of a limp.

Mindless conformity is behind many of the ways in which we give up free will. Take a famous example in social psychology called the Asch conformity experiment.[2] People were shown three lines of different lengths and their task was to declare which of these lines was the same length as one of the other lines they were shown. Unbeknownst to the participants, accomplices working with the experimenter were planted to intentionally give an obviously wrong answer before it was the participants' turn to respond. Typically, the participants conformed and repeated the wrong answer that the person ahead of them had given rather than point out the error. We see this kind of thing all around us. Two of your friends refuse to take the Covid vaccine. While you thought the vaccine could be a good thing, do you now have second thoughts and delay getting it? Similarly, imagine you weren't inclined to get the vaccine but two of your good friends got it. Just as the participants in the Asch study went along with others despite what they initially saw, we too often conform.

Accepting certainty is the most flagrant instance of unnecessarily limiting our free will. As soon as we think we know something, we stop considering other, potentially better alternatives. Hence the expression, "Frequently in error but rarely in doubt." Our mindless acceptance of certainty robs us of the freedom of choice.

We live in a world governed by the principles of science. The precision with which we can now measure the world around us, however, is only as useful as the degree of mindfulness we employ to analyze it. Our measures and tools are context-limited and subjective regardless of the objectivity we try to impart to them. Science becomes mindless when we conflate precision with certainty. Scientific evidence can only yield probabilities, but too often we take these probabilities and convert them into absolutes, making it hard for us to question basic assumptions.

I experienced this many years ago when we knew little about dementia. My idea was that senility, as it was then called, might be a mindful response to an overly routinized environment. Yes, you didn't misread it. I'm saying there may have been an advantage to senility. That is, some of the bizarre things senile people say and do may be a mindful relief from all the redundancy they undergo. Which would be better, living a life on automatic pilot or having bizarre novel thoughts? Surely, I reasoned, senility is socially maladaptive. It makes those around us uncomfortable. But if the novel thoughts were understood as a result of being mindful, given that we've already found that mindfulness leads to longevity, the crazy thoughts could be biologically adaptive. *That is, could those who were diagnosed as senile and perhaps constantly seeing the world anew, actually live longer?*

To test this idea, many years ago my then student Pearl Beck and my colleagues Ronnie Janoff-Bulman, Christine

Timko, and I collected data on people who, in addition to having heart disease, were labeled senile or not.[3] We found that those labeled senile lived significantly longer than those who only had heart disease. This was 1984. When we submitted the research paper to a major scientific journal, it was soundly rejected. The categorical reason for the rejection was that the "journal didn't publish research in progress." That is, they wanted to publish only papers that presented final answers, proof in numbers. Without any previous research suggesting anything positive about senility, the journal editors assumed there couldn't be any advantages from senility; ours was, therefore, research in progress, not definitive. I found—and still find—this response irrational. Everything in science is "in progress." There are no final answers; we are always learning new things about the mindful body. (We eventually published the paper in the *Academic Psychology Bulletin.*)

Many diseases are labeled as chronic, and chronic is understood to be incurable. If a disease is deemed to be incurable, we would be foolish to try to cure it. *Yet no science can prove incurability.* All science can prove is that what was tried didn't work at the time for the people on whom it was tried. That is, whether or not it can be cured is indeterminate, and indeterminate is quite different from uncontrollable. Moreover, people who self-heal are usually missing from medical experiments. And, as stated before, many people self-heal without even knowing they were sick in the first place. In any experiment, the researcher must make many hidden decisions regarding the parameters of the study (who the participants are, the time and circumstances in which they'll be tested, the amount of the independent variable to administer, and so forth). With these parameters out of sight, findings regarding impossibility may seem more sure and more general than they might otherwise be. This is why I tend to design my research to uncover what is possible rather than rule out something as impossible. Most of the time, we are looking for what might be rather than what is.

People tend to seek certainty but by unwittingly accepting the status quo, we cease to notice change. We always put on our glasses to help us see and become blind to the conditions under which we could see well without them. We go to a therapist who offers us a different way to look at a situation and, rather than realizing there are many possible alternatives, too often we accept this understanding now as our new reality. That is, if we think we know, we have no doubt. If we have no doubt, we have no choice. Given that our experience is constantly changing and that everything looks different from different perspectives, unwittingly we're giving up benefits that we don't even know about. The negative effects can be widespread. Accepting the status quo by definition limits innovation.

We may not be living in a completely mindless dystopia, but we nevertheless experience far more mindlessness than most of us realize.

What changes for us in a mindful utopia? Importantly, mind-body unity suggests that we do not have to be slaves to our passions, victims of addictions, or controlled by primes or cues in the environment. We become the masters of our fates. In some sense, health may be only a thought away.

In a mindful utopia we would stop being judgmental and recognize that behavior makes sense to the actor from their perspective. The discomfort we feel when we're being judged would evaporate and we'd be willing to try new things without concern for what we're "supposed to do" or what everyone else is doing. This would result in a massive decrease in the amount of stress we'd experience. And with less stress comes better health.

It might be worth a moment to consider what life would be like if we weren't ruled by scarcity worries. If we lived in a world of plenty, social comparisons, predictions, and decisions would become unimportant, and rules would not be meaningful constraints. If you always wanted what you got, it wouldn't matter what decisions you made, and if your decisions didn't matter, there would be no need for predictions. We make social comparisons to see who is more worthy of limited resources, so in our world of plenty, they too would fall by the wayside. With scarcity worries gone, rigid rules would become merely conventions. We develop rules to keep people in place. People typically break rules so they can get what they want. If they always wanted what they got anyway, rule breaking would become unnecessary.

The most important presumed scarce resource is healthcare. As we have seen, our health is largely governed by our psychology, thus good health is available to us all.

Although we often associate a utopia with perfection, to create a mindful utopia we would need in some way to do away with the static notion of perfection. Maybe it would be better to replace perfection with the idea of uncertain expectations. Expectations about the future would still be encouraged, but we would feel free to adjust and change our expectations to fit our current circumstances. Perfection would be the full acceptance of uncertainty.

Consider our schools. Why do people believe learning must be tedious, hard, and rarely enjoyable? Our research has shown that mindful learning gives us energy and is fun. We can gamify academic subject matter, or we can simply teach mindful learning, which makes memorizing obsolete. Having difficulty memorizing is a health hazard because it is stressful. Moreover, in mindful schools, there would be no winners and losers. As a result, again, there would be less stress. The particulars of how to do this are not as important as the belief that it should be done.

And what about in the business context? In the business world there's too often an unquestioned assumption that to get anything done people need to be told what to do. On the contrary, in a study that orchestra conductor Timothy Russell, my student Noah Eisenkraft, and I ran, we found this is not always the case.[4] In our experiment, we instructed some orchestras (which are businesses, even if not in the strictest sense) to be mindful and make their performances subtly new each time they played. In contrast, we instructed other orchestras to replicate past performances with which they were pleased, and we defined this as playing mindlessly. We taped the performances and played the recordings for people unaware of the study. The results showed a strong preference for the mindful performances. When writing these results up for publication, it occurred to me that the findings suggested some novel advice for leaders. We found that when everyone was being mindful, doing their own thing, and actively noticing new things about the music, a superior coordinated performance resulted. Perhaps the primary job of the leader, just as with teachers, is to encourage the mindfulness of those being led or taught.

Similarly, if we relax our conventional ideas about job qualifications, many exciting possibilities may await us. In a sense, no one has the right experience for any particular job. Teachers are trained for yesterday not tomorrow. The CEO of a multinational company will be running a company that is different than the company was before they took charge. If you are hiring teachers and employees, you might have better success by mindfully adjusting tomorrow's tasks to suit their strengths than to mindlessly hire people whose strengths match yesterday's tasks. Everyone brings something to the table. The larger point is that by creating mindful schools and businesses, we learn how to avoid using yesterday's solutions to solve today's problems. With greater success comes less stress, and with less stress comes better health.

A NEW APPROACH TO HEALTH

Decades ago, I was a consultant to a nursing home. I carried around a clipboard to signal my official status since I wasn't wearing a white coat. After a while, I saw I never used it but brought it anyway to establish my status. When I realized this, I left it home. I felt that whatever respect I was to garner had to be based on my current behavior rather than my credentials. I was surprised to see how much more the visits meant to me and how much more I got out of them after I dropped the props associated with "researcher/consultant" and simply spent time there as a human being.

In the same way, I think that medical professionals should be in uniform only when they are performing a medical procedure; this would make them far more approachable when stopping by the bedside. And their individual humanity would take the place of mindlessly assuming a medical role. Under these circumstances, positive relationships between staff and patients may be more likely to flourish.

In a mindful utopia, medical professionals would do more than just change their clothes. They'd be taught to attend to the variability in their patients' symptoms, demeanor, and overall well-being. Because attending to variability keeps everyone mindful and engaged, it stands to reason that burnout for doctors and nurses would be reduced. And patients who interact with more mindful staff would likely feel more confident that their voices were being heard. Probably most important, by attending to variability, medical professionals would use information about changes to improve patient care and the speed of recovery.

Patients should also be taught to be active members in their own wellness and to be more mindful generally, not only with respect to symptom variability. Given the importance of choice in maintaining a healthy life, patients need to understand that they are full partners in the care of their health.

If asked, "What would a mindful utopia feel like?" perhaps most important, we would experience the positive effects of the capacity to change our minds, create options and decide among them, and live with control and ownership over our lives.

As the general public's awareness of mindfulness was growing, it was bound to happen that someone would try to gain fame by disparaging it. Thus, I was not surprised when a journalist who was interviewing me asked me if mindfulness is just a fad. My response was, "If every day you make toast and burn it in the process and someone shows you that all you need to do is change the dial on your toaster, would you go back to burning your toast after a while?" Once we learn to do something that helps, it's not a fad; it becomes a way of life.

MINDFUL MEDICINE

Medical errors are legion. This may not be surprising when we realize that no matter how bright and caring they are, physicians are people and people make mistakes. On any given day, nurses and doctors may not have had enough sleep, or may be stressed or preoccupied with personal matters. And perhaps most important, people are frequently mindless. Bestselling author and social psychologist Robert Cialdini tells of a case where a nurse was instructed to "give the medicine in the R-ear." She read it as rear end rather than right ear.[5]

There are many ways medical education, whether for doctors or nurses, unintentionally encourages mindlessness. Learned facts are often regarded as unchanging and absolute, there is little tolerance for doubt or uncertainty, and patients are categorized according to preconceived schemas and groupings. Medical doctor Shahar Arzy of Geneva University Hospitals and her colleagues conducted a study showing that when doctors are given just one misleading detail it can lead them down the wrong path in making their diagnosis.[6] They gave a group of internists ten vignettes regarding medical problems and asked them to make a diagnosis. In each vignette there was a misleading detail. For example, a young girl who had a ski accident complains of pain. Her pain was due to non-Hodgkin's lymphoma, and the data available to them clearly indicated this. But because of the misleading detail about the ski accident, they misdiagnosed her. Over the course of the study, the presence of the misleading detail resulted in a misdiagnosis 90 percent of the time. Again, when people are mindless, they are frequently in error but rarely in doubt. Perhaps physicians, like the rest of us, would be more effective if they accepted uncertainty as the rule, rather than the exception. When we know we don't know we are more attuned to the present situation.

Doctor and author Atul Gawande has been at the forefront of ways to reduce medical errors. He pioneered surgical checklists to ensure that surgical teams follow standard procedures and don't mindlessly overlook small details that could be costly to patient health.[7] In advance of every procedure the team is required to go over a checklist and to confirm important details such as whether a patient had been given antibiotics before any incision was made to decrease the likelihood of postsurgical infection. To date, Gawande has collected data on about one thousand procedures in eight hospitals and has found that the use of checklists reduced errors by an impressive 50 percent.

But of course, checklists don't always ensure mindfulness. Indeed, when the questions on a checklist become too familiar, we may stop paying attention. When I complete a checklist at the airport about what I've packed, after the first two or three questions, it often becomes clear that the answer is "no," so I don't feel I need to read the rest very carefully. No, I did not have anyone watch my suitcase for me in the airport. No, there are no weapons in my suitcase, and so on.

Instead of checklists to which we answer yes or no, what might happen if a more nuanced response was required? For example, instead of asking "Is the patient alert?," what if the question was "How alert is the patient?" Medical staff would probably look at the patient more carefully to make this assessment. Even questions like "How dilated are the patient's pupils?" would lead to closer inspection.

MENTAL HEALTH

Even if the questions can be answered on a more continuous scale rather than simply yes or no, checklists presume we know what to look for, and they make it necessary to measure responses based on preconceived notions. Sometimes the better approach might be to collect raw, uncategorized data, and see what new things we can learn from it, rather than squeeze it into old categories. One of the most promising areas for this kind of approach is in mental health.

It's not an exaggeration to say that when mental illness goes undiagnosed it poses a significant health risk for the depressed person, as well as his or her family, neighbors, and coworkers. Yet it is expensive, time-consuming, and often inaccurate to do in-person screenings to identify people at risk. Even more, mental health may not fit neatly into prepackaged categories.

When he was my student, Andrew Reece's PhD thesis was

designed to see if he could identify predictive markers of mental illness in social media data.[8] He began by scanning and interpreting text and images posted on Twitter and Instagram to see if it was possible to identify people at risk of depression and PTSD. He looked at an enormous amount of data— 279,951 Twitter posts and 43,950 Instagram posts—and used color analysis, face detection, semantic analysis, and natural language processing to identify features of the posted photos and texts that might help predict depression. We can think of all of these approaches as trying to find new and hidden yet consistent patterns in the raw data (photos and texts) rather than trying to categorize the raw data into predetermined diagnostic categories.

Ultimately, with the help of his computer, Andrew's model was able to differentiate between healthy and depressed individuals and was as good or better than general practitioners' ability to make successful category-based diagnoses. This was true even when he limited his analysis to social media content posted before the first diagnosis of depression. In the case of the Twitter data, it was clear that depression could be diagnosed several months prior to a clinician's diagnosis.

Imagine the advantages of early screening and detection of mental illness. If we caught it early enough, suffering could be drastically reduced, and perhaps hospital care would become unnecessary. Of course, there's always the possibility we would start to mindlessly rely on computer programs written at an earlier time when different information may have been relevant, which means human intervention would never become unnecessary.

MINDFUL HOSPITALS

While at present most people in the medical world may disagree with my view that stress is the number one killer, it would be hard to find many who don't think that stress is bad for our health. Nevertheless, there is little focus on how to make hospitals, or more generally the administration of medical treatment, less stressful. We have to go to the hospital, say, for a mammogram or chest X-ray, or because we broke our collarbone, or for a hundred other reasons. Hospitals ostensibly are for healing, yet as we enter the building we're likely to get sicker because our overwhelming feeling is fear. Moreover, our attention may be drawn to those who are in worse shape than we are who may seem to represent our future selves. The environment is sterile, and medical personnel quickly walk the halls with serious facial expressions, again conveying gloom and doom. This is clearly not a place we want to be.

Perhaps this makes sense in the ICU, but it is of questionable wisdom for the rest of the hospital. On the other hand, the children's ward is often made to be colorful and light-hearted. Colorfulness and joy don't mean that our ailment is not in need of serious care. If you are dealing with cancer as an adult, your surroundings in a hospital are quite distinct from what you would experience as a child with cancer. At what age would we want to give up an uplifting environment for a stressful one?

What would a mindful hospital look like? I think these would be places where people worry less about disease and dying and instead learn how to live.

For starters, patients' families and significant others would be involved in all aspects of their care. In my experience, significant others too often feel helpless in the typical hospital setting when instead they could be of great help. When my mother was in the hospital, it would have been comforting and reassuring for both her and me if I could have, at the least, wheeled her gurney to the X-ray room. But, for insurance reasons, this wasn't allowed. We had to wait for a seventeen-year-old staff member to move her there instead.

By understanding the importance of keeping family close by, the hospital could partner with childcare groups so that parents wouldn't need to worry about their children when they're in the hospital but could also see them when it was important to do so.

A mindful hospital would recognize the importance of relationships with people undergoing similar health issues. Patients would therefore be given the choice to participate in various group activities. These might involve gentle chair yoga, meditation, mindfulness exercises, card games, and discussion groups. Thus, rather than being kept from one another, the patient would be encouraged right from the start to form friendships and find ways to be helpful to one another. As I've mentioned, a good deal of social psychological research has found how important social support is for our health.

We know how important the physical environment can be to well-being, so a mindful hospital would be full of color. It would resemble a spa as much as a health facility. Mindful hospitals would encourage people to think about being outside of the hospital, and would connect them to gardens, sitting rooms, and kitchens. Indeed, in one study, Roger Ulrich, former professor at the Centre for Healthcare Architecture at Chalmers University of Technology in Sweden, found that people assigned to hospital rooms with windows overlooking gardens healed faster and needed fewer painkillers than people whose rooms faced a brick wall.[9]

The mission of the mindful hospital would be to stretch the possibilities of health and healing dynamically and continuously. The goal of every staff member would be to encourage patients to add more life to one's years, and not just more years to one's life.

UNIMPOSSIBLE

Almost thirty years ago, encouraged by a friend, I thought it would be fun to go to an iridologist. Iridology is an alternative to traditional medicine in which the characteristics of the iris are used to reveal aspects of our health. Until my friend mentioned it, I had no idea that iridology even existed, but I became curious to learn more about it. The iridologist took a picture of the iris of my eye and then told me I had a small gall bladder problem. As it happened, one week before I'd gone to the doctor because of a stubborn pain I thought was in my stomach. He said I had a gallstone and prescribed broth, gelatin, and rest for the week. I was amazed that the iridologist caught this from a photo of my eye. Given everything I've laid out in this book, it won't surprise you that this no longer strikes me as incredible. I believe that everything present in our bodies on any level is present on every level; we just don't have the tools yet to see it or the awareness that we should even look.

Powerful mindsets inhibit our ability even in the simplest of situations. The now-famous invisible gorilla study conducted by Dan Simons and Chris Chabris when they were at Harvard is a good example. In their study, participants watched a video of people playing basketball, and during the game a person in a gorilla suit came onto the court.[10] Amazingly, most people watching the video don't see the gorilla. After Dan showed this at a colloquium at Harvard, we ran a pilot study to see who *did* notice the gorilla. One group was first given instructions to be mindful. "You are going to see a video of a basketball game. All basketball games are like all other basketball games in some ways, which is why they are called basketball games. But just as certainly, each game is different. While you watch the video, please notice how it is the same and how it is different." Another group simply watched the video without instructions. Most of the participants given the mindfulness instructions saw the gorilla.

Dan and Chris's study was a far more elaborate version of an experiment I described in chapter 9. When we presented people with an index card that had familiar phrases with repeated words, most people did not see the repeated words. They didn't see them even when we offered them money for being correct or when we asked them to tell us how many words were on the card. People who had just finished meditating, by contrast, saw the repeated word, and those in the presence of someone mindful did as well.

This blindness also exists in science. Itai Yanai of the Institute for Computational Medicine at NYU and Martin Lercher, head of the Computational Cell Biology research group at Heinrich Heine University in Germany, found that when their participants had strong hypotheses, they would miss what otherwise was in plain sight.[11] That is, we tend to find what we're looking for and miss the rest of what's there to be seen. Participants were to analyze a data set for a study purportedly concerning body mass index for 1,786 people and the number of steps they took in a day. They plotted the data set, one dot for each person. The finished graph depicted a gorilla. The participants who came to the experiment with a focused hypothesis were less likely to see the image. The stronger our expectations, the more blind we become. Thus, it is not surprising that, when doctors read a patient's chart, they can lock into it and miss important information if they are not prompted to be mindful.

Sometimes our mindsets don't blind us to what otherwise would be visible but set us up for other kinds of trouble. Psychologist Dan Wegner[12] found that, when instructed not to think about something—say, a white bear—no matter how hard we try, it still comes back to mind. This has come to be known as "the white bear effect."

It occurred to me that the effect may occur only with people who have a preconceived notion about a bear. My students and I tested this by showing one group of people a single white bear while showing another group four different-looking white bears—thin, fat, old, or young—before we gave them the instruction "Don't think of a white bear." For the latter group, it would be unclear which white bear not to think about; they now had a choice and were mindful. Only the first group had trouble following that instruction. The relevance of this finding to our health is that we can control our thoughts more than we realize. Rather than try not to think about something, such as whether cancer is incurable or diabetes can't be managed, we'd be better off thinking about it differently. We can choose how to think about things. By re-thinking, or reframing a thought from different angles, we can achieve a new level of personal control.

CHAPTER 11

A Mindful Utopia

You were born with wings.
Why prefer to crawl through life?
—RUMI

When nothing is certain, isn't virtually everything possible? Whether it is George Bernard Shaw's Eliza Doolittle, a Cockney flower girl whom Henry Higgins helps transform into a woman of high society, or Rocky Balboa, a small-time boxer who becomes a world champion, we have countless examples of the possibility of major change in our culture. They are the subjects of many of our favorite stories. But as much as we believe in stories of transformation, we tend not to believe that transformation is for us.

Most conscious thought deals with rigidly understood pre-packaged information. Aging is solely a time of loss, some of us are just worth more than others, and chronic illnesses can't be cured. Living mindfully allows us to see past these thoughts and see the possibility for chronic health. As a result, it enhances access to all those new possibilities we typically neglect.

Indeed, there is a fair amount of data showing that with a little effort, people of any age can perform at a higher level than they currently do in most every respect. In Robert Rosenthal and Lenore Jacobson's important 1968 study on the Pygmalion effect, changing teachers' expectations for students was shown to make exceptional students out of those for whom there was no reason to believe they were special.[1] Elementary school students were chosen at random, and their teachers were told they were essentially diamonds in the rough, priming the expectation that these students had hidden talents that perhaps the teacher could draw out and help develop. By the end of the school year, the students significantly improved their IQ scores. Planting the idea of possibility changes outcomes, not unlike the way in which placebos work. But still, we lead most students to believe they just don't have what it takes.

Too often we think we're doing the best we can. But we're not, not even close. Our expectations for ourselves and one another are too often woefully low. I believe this is true regarding our physical abilities, our sensibilities, our health, and our cognitive prowess. If I score 30 out of 100 on a test of ability, and then score 50 out of 100, progress is easy to see. But if I do worse on the second test, why would I believe that I can succeed if I have a rigid expectation that success typically unfolds in a straight line? Success typically does not unfold in a straight line. We do better and then not so well and then if we continue, we often do even better.

The judgments we face aren't simply confined to test taking. The quality of our ideas is also judged, but by what standards? We're often pulled down to the norm, derided if we see the world differently from others. Galileo threatened the prevailing worldview and was judged to be a heretic, sentenced to life imprisonment. Few ideas are as earthshaking as his, and yet many of us are still afraid to think differently and thus remain imprisoned by our mindlessness.

We're taught these limits early in life. Parents, teachers, and our culture reinforce these low expectations. You're not able to drink at age sixteen because you're not wise enough to know when you've had enough. If you enjoy gambling at casinos, be careful you don't become addicted. What these warnings and restrictions have in common is a focus on prevention. True, if the sixteen-year-old doesn't drink at all, the problem won't occur. And if adults don't gamble, they won't become addicted. But is this the most effective way to create a culture? I think not. I think it may be better to learn from the sixteen-year-olds who are able to drink modestly or the adults who can enjoy an evening at a casino and not lose control. Rather than teach from the bottom or to the norm, perhaps we should start by looking at successes and assume that their success is available to the rest of us in meaningful ways. Presently when we find that some people are far better than most of us at something, we label them as "super": super tasters, super smellers, talented, superior learners. This suggests that the rest of us cannot possibly do as well. But we can't know that that is the case.

Before we conducted the counterclockwise study, for example, I knew that most people believed eyesight worsens with age. Some might acknowledge that there are outliers for whom this isn't true, but the norm said it was true and biologically determined. Nevertheless, we conducted the study with "ordinary," not extraordinary, adults and found that vision can improve—an important lesson for a good number of us.

By embodying their younger selves, the men in the counterclockwise study showed that seniors are capable of far more than typically believed. Is this also true for younger people? If younger people embodied their future selves—clockwise rather than counterclockwise—would they behave with the acumen and sensibility of their future older selves even in situations for which they are considered too immature? My lab members and I believe this but haven't put it to the test. We also believe they could do this without giving up the mindfulness endemic to being young.

When taken together, the completed studies I've presented in this book suggest that much of what we have assumed was impossible may actually be available to us now: Vision and hearing can be improved, symptoms from chronic illness can be abetted, and we can become less stressed, less judgmental, and happier among other things, without intensive training or cost.

No matter what our age, more is possible. As my friend and entertainer Zoe Lewis sings, "Don't stop playing just because you've grown old, or you'll grow old because you've stopped your play.... You're never too old to be young.... When they tell you to act your age, they're obviously lacking in expertise. Can't they see it doesn't matter unless you're a bottle of wine or you're a piece of cheese? So when those twilight years smile down like diamonds upon you, please remember when you think you've done it all, you're gonna always find something new."

It doesn't matter if we're old or young, life can be lived fully without hesitation. We can choose to be whatever age we want at any moment. Why wait?

As more people come to appreciate and exploit the power of uncertainty, a mindful utopia may be closer than many think. Once we recognize that mindless decisions from the past are limiting us, there is little stopping us from redesigning the world to better fit our current needs rather than using yesterday to determine today and tomorrow. When we do this, that which was previously taken as impossible may yield to a new possibility. Isn't it time to unexpect everything so we can each be the hero of our own story?

In our current world, we presume scarcity and that we're unable to be on top. We see we are unable to take the risks that "they" are able to take, and making important decisions is just not our forte. We're simply not on the tail end of the normal distribution. This way of thinking has led to a vertical society where we're constantly comparing to see who is better or worse than we are.

Once we question the foundational aspects of our behavior, the vertical can become horizontal. Yes, we are each different from one another but not in the absolute sense of better and worse.

I wrote a little song for my grandkids, Emmett and Theo, when they were five years old to the tune of an old Sara Lee commercial. It's not a great composition and you're probably fortunate that you're reading the words rather than hearing me sing them. Nevertheless, I sing it all the time—even to my students—because I think the underlying idea is so important. It goes like this:

Everyone doesn't know something. But everyone knows
   something else.
Everyone can't do something. But everyone can do
   something else.

One day when we were in the car Theo started whistling. I said, "Theo, you're such a good whistler," at which point his brother, Emmett, said, "Grandma El, I was learning something else while Theo was learning how to whistle." Hopefully, they'll never feel less than anyone else, and a mindful body will greet their older selves.

Acknowledgments

The Mindful Body went through many iterations, and so there are many people to whom I am grateful. When this book started out as a memoir, I sought the wisdom of several extraordinary writer friends, among them Dominique Browning, Laurie Hays, Pamela Painter, and Phyllis Katz, to see if I was disclosing too many of my private adventures, and to see if other stories were sufficiently interesting to include.

On the advice of my dear friend David Miller, who worked with me on *The Power of Mindful Learning; On Becoming an Artist: Reinventing Yourself Through Mindful Creativity;* and *Counterclockwise: Mindful Health and the Power of Possibility,* the book became an idea memoir, which seemed better suited to reconsider ideas from my past and to present new ideas.

New ideas came rushing forth and took over, and my idea memoir became the current book. Endless discussions with my respected colleagues, friends, and lab members Philip Maymin and Stu Albert helped make the journey to the present exciting and fruitful. They may be the only people I have met whose ideas are more extreme than my own. I'm especially grateful to my very dear friend and scholar Lenore Weitzman, who painstakingly commented on almost every sentence in the manuscript.

I thank the members of my lab—faculty, postdocs, and graduate and undergraduate students past and present, many of whom are now professors running their own labs. They are always the most important players in expanding and refining my research. Most important regarding *The Mindful Body* are John Allman, Peter Aungle, Colin Bosma, Stayce Camparo, Benzion Chanowitz, Jaewoo Chung, Matt Cohen, Alia Crum, Laura Delizonna, Maja Djkic, Michelle Dow, Noah Eisenkraft, Mohsen Fatemi, Adam Grant, Karyn Gunnet-Shoval, Chiara Haller, Laura Hsu, Andrew Kiruluta, Ren Koa, Becca Levy, Clayton McClintock, Mihnea Moldoveanu, Christelle Ngnoumen, Kris Nichols, Jay Olson, Ozgun Atasoy, Francesco Pagnini, Deborah Phillips, Andrew Reece, Dasha Sandra, Wendy Smith, Loralyn Thompson, John Welch, Judith White, Ryan Williams, and Leeat Yariv.

I'm truly grateful to Jonah Lehrer, Lisa Adams, and my Random House editor, Marnie Cochran, whose editorial acumen helped shape the book. Finally, I want to thank Merloyd Lawrence, with whom I first worked on *Mindfulness*. A remarkable editor and dear friend, it was she before her recent death who tried to tame me when she thought I had stepped too far from what many see as impossible.

As the memoir draft of this book made clear, having an extremely supportive family then and now has enabled me, for better or worse, to think differently and to think about how to create a world of plenty for everyone. To each of them I extend my gratitude and love.

Notes

INTRODUCTION

1. Ellen J. Langer, *Mindfulness* (Reading, Mass.: Addison-Wesley, 1989).
2. Ellen J. Langer, *Counterclockwise: Mindful Health and the Power of Possibility* (New York: Ballantine Books, 2009).

CHAPTER 1: WHOSE RULES?

1. Russell H. Fazio, Edwin A. Effrein, and Victoria J. Falender, "Self-Perceptions Following Social Interaction," *Journal of Personality and Social Psychology* 41, no. 2 (1981): 232.
2. Alison L. Chasteen et al., "How Feelings of Stereotype Threat Influence Older Adults' Memory Performance," *Experimental Aging Research* 31, no. 3 (2005): 235–60.
3. Steven J. Spencer, Claude M. Steele, and Diane M. Quinn, "Stereotype Threat and Women's Math Performance," *Journal of Experimental Social Psychology* 35, no. 1 (1999): 4–28.
4. Christelle Tchangha Ngnoumen, "The Use of Socio-Cognitive Mindfulness in Mitigating Implicit Bias and Stereotype-Activated Behaviors," PhD diss., Harvard University, 2019.
5. Anthony G. Greenwald, Brian A. Nosek, and Mahzarin R. Banaji, "Understanding and Using the Implicit Association Test: I. An Improved Scoring Algorithm," *Journal of Personality and Social Psychology* 85, no. 2 (2003): 197.
6. Ellen J. Langer, *On Becoming an Artist: Reinventing Yourself Through Mindful Creativity* (New York: Ballantine Books, 2007).

7. Peter Aungle, Karyn Gunnet-Shoval, and Ellen J. Langer, "The Border-line Effect for Diabetes: When No Difference Makes a Difference," unpublished manuscript.

CHAPTER 2: RISK, PREDICTION, AND THE ILLUSION OF CONTROL

1. Michael W. Morris, Erica Carranza, and Craig R. Fox, "Mistaken Identity: Activating Conservative Political Identities Induces 'Conservative' Financial Decisions," *Psychological Science* 19, no. 11 (2008): 1154–60.
2. Daniel Gilbert, *Stumbling on Happiness* (Toronto: Vintage Canada, 2009).
3. Ellen J. Langer, "The Illusion of Control," *Journal of Personality and Social Psychology* 32, no. 2 (1975): 311.
4. Nathanael J. Fast et al., "Illusory Control: A Generative Force Behind Power's Far-Reaching Effects," *Psychological Science* 20, no. 4 (2009): 502–8.
5. Mark Fenton-O'Creevy et al., "Trading on Illusions: Unrealistic Perceptions of Control and Trading Performance," *Journal of Occupational and Organizational Psychology* 76, no. 1 (2003): 53–68.
6. David C. Glass and Jerome E. Singer, *Urban Stress: Experiments on Noise and Social Stressors* (New York: Academic Press, 1972).

CHAPTER 3: A WORLD OF PLENTY

1. S. Snow and E. Langer, unpublished data.
2. Ellen J. Langer, *Mindfulness,* Twenty-Fifth Anniversary Edition (New York: Da Capo Press, 2014).
3. Mark Twain, *The Prince and the Pauper* (New York: Bantam Dell, 2007).
4. Raymond Queneau, *Exercises in Style* (London: John Colder, 1998).
5. Mihnea Moldoveanu and Ellen Langer, "False Memories of the Future: A Critique of the Applications of Probabilistic Reasoning to the Study of Cognitive Processes," *Psychological Review* 109, no. 2 (2002): 358.
6. Ellen Langer et al., "Believing Is Seeing: Using Mindlessness (Mindfully) to Improve Visual Acuity," *Psychological Science* 21, no. 5 (2010): 661–66.

CHAPTER 4: WHY DECIDE?

1. Irving L. Janis and Leon Mann, *Decision Making: A Psychological Analysis of Conflict, Choice, and Commitment* (New York: Free Press, 1977).
2. Daniel Kahneman, *Thinking, Fast and Slow* (New York: Macmillan, 2011).
3. H. Igor Ansoff, *Corporate Strategy: An Analytic Approach to Business Policy for Growth and Expansion* (New York: McGraw-Hill, 1965).
4. Barry Schwartz, *The Paradox of Choice: Why More Is Less* (New York: Ecco, 2004).
5. Herbert A. Simon, "Rational Choice and the Structure of the Environment," *Psychological Review* 63, no. 2 (1956): 129.
6. Clyde Hendrick, Judson Mills, and Charles A. Kiesler, "Decision Time

as a Function of the Number and Complexity of Equally Attractive Alternatives," *Journal of Personality and Social Psychology* 8, no. 3p1 (1968): 313.

7. Sheena S. Iyengar and Mark R. Lepper, "When Choice Is Demotivating: Can One Desire Too Much of a Good Thing?" *Journal of Personality and Social Psychology* 79, no. 6 (2000): 995.

8. Martin Lindstrom, *Buyology: Truth and Lies About Why We Buy* (New York: Currency, 2008).

9. Sian L. Beilock and Thomas H. Carr, "When High-Powered People Fail: Working Memory and 'Choking Under Pressure' in Math," *Psychological Science* 16, no. 2 (2005): 101–5.

10. Shai Danziger, Jonathan Levav, and Liora Avnaim-Pesso, "Extraneous Factors in Judicial Decisions," *Proceedings of the National Academy of Sciences* 108, no. 17 (2011): 6889–92.

11. Daniel Kahneman and Amos Tversky, "Prospect Theory: An Analysis of Decision Under Risk," in L. C. MacLean and W. T. Ziemba, *Handbook of the Fundamentals of Financial Decision Making: Part I* (Hackensack, N.J.: World Scientific, 2013), 99–127.

12. Antonio R. Damasio, *Descartes' Error* (New York: Random House, 2006).

13. Simon, "Rational Choice."

CHAPTER 5: LEVEL UP

1. Judith B. White et al., "Frequent Social Comparisons and Destructive Emotions and Behaviors: The Dark Side of Social Comparisons," *Journal of Adult Development* 13, no. 1 (2006): 36–44.

2. Leon Festinger, "A Theory of Social Comparison Processes," *Human Relations* 7, no. 2 (1954): 117–40.

3. William J. McGuire, "An Additional Future for Psychological Science," *Perspectives on Psychological Science* 8, no. 4 (2013): 414–23.

4. Samuel Rickless, *Plato's Form in Transition: A Reading of the Parmenides* (Cambridge: Cambridge University Press, 2007).

5. Kristopher L. Nichols, Neha Dhawan, and Ellen J. Langer, "Try Versus Do: The Framing Effects of Language on Performance," in preparation.

CHAPTER 6: MIND AND BODY AS ONE

1. George L. Engel, "The Clinical Application of the Biopsychosocial Model," *The Journal of Medicine and Philosophy: A Forum for Bioethics and Philosophy of Medicine* 6, no. 2 (1981): 101–24.

2. Judith Rodin and Ellen J. Langer, "Long-term Effects of a Control-Relevant Intervention with the Institutionalized Aged," *Journal of Personality and Social Psychology* 35, no. 12 (1977): 897.

3. Richard Schulz and Barbara H. Hanusa, "Long-term Effects of Control and Predictability-Enhancing Interventions: Findings and Ethical Issues," *Journal of Personality and Social Psychology* 36, no. 11 (1978): 1194.

4. Ellen J. Langer et al., "Environmental Determinants of Memory Improvement in Late Adulthood," *Journal of Personality and Social Psychology* 37, no. 11 (1979): 2003.

5. Charles N. Alexander et al., "Transcendental Meditation, Mindfulness, and Longevity: An Experimental Study with the Elderly," *Journal of Personality and Social Psychology* 57, no. 6 (1989): 950.

6. Maya Schiller, Tamar L. Ben-Shaanan, and Asya Rolls, "Neuronal Regulation of Immunity: Why, How and Where?" *Nature Reviews Immunology* 21, no. 1 (2021): 20–36.

7. Esther Landhuis, "The Brain Can Recall and Reawaken Past Immune Responses," *Quanta Magazine*, November 8, 2021, https://www.quanta magazine.org/new-science-shows-immune-memory-in-the-brain -20211108/.

8. Tamar L. Ben-Shaanan et al., "Activation of the Reward System Boosts Innate and Adaptive Immunity," *Nature Medicine* 22, no. 8 (2016): 940–44.

9. E. Langer, B. Chanowitz, S., Jacobs, M. Rhodes, M., Palmerino, and P. Thayer, "Nonsequential Development and Aging," in eds. C. Alexander and E. Langer, *Higher Stages of Human Development* (New York: Oxford University Press, 1990).

10. Francesco Pagnini et al., "Ageing as a Mindset: A Study Protocol to Rejuvenate Older Adults with a Counterclockwise Psychological Intervention," *BMJ Open* 9, no. 7 (2019): e030411.

11. Laura M. Hsu, Jaewoo Chung, and Ellen J. Langer, "The Influence of Age-Related Cues on Health and Longevity," *Perspectives on Psychological Science* 5, no. 6 (2010): 632–48.

12. Alia J. Crum and Ellen J. Langer, "Mind-Set Matters: Exercise and the Placebo Effect," *Psychological Science* 18, no. 2 (2007): 165–71.

13. Octavia H. Zahrt and Alia J. Crum, "Perceived Physical Activity and Mortality: Evidence from Three Nationally Representative US Samples," *Health Psychology* 36, no. 11 (2017): 1017.

14. Abiola Keller et al., "Does the Perception That Stress Affects Health Matter? The Association with Health and Mortality," *Health Psychology* 31, no. 5 (2012): 677.

15. Shadab A. Rahman et al., "Manipulating Sleep Duration Perception Changes Cognitive Performance: An Exploratory Analysis," *Journal of Psychosomatic Research* 132 (2020): 109992.

16. Langer, *Counterclockwise*, 123.

17. Stayce Camparo et al., "The Fatigue Illusion: The Physical Effects of Mindlessness," *Humanities and Social Sciences Communications*, in review.

18. Bradley P. Turnwald et al., "Learning One's Genetic Risk Changes Physiology Independent of Actual Genetic Risk," *Nature Human Behaviour* 3, no. 1 (2019): 48–56.

19. Lawrence E. Williams and John A. Bargh, "Experiencing Physical

Warmth Promotes Interpersonal Warmth," *Science* 322, no. 5901 (2008): 606–7.

20. Hans Ijzerman and Gün R. Semin, "The Thermometer of Social Relations: Mapping Social Proximity on Temperature," *Psychological Science* 20, no. 10 (2009): 1214–20.

21. Tristen K. Inagaki and Naomi I. Eisenberger, "Shared Neural Mechanisms Underlying Social Warmth and Physical Warmth," *Psychological Science* 24, no. 11 (2013): 2272–80.

22. Naomi I. Eisenberger, Matthew D. Lieberman, and Kipling D. Williams, "Does Rejection Hurt? An fMRI Study of Social Exclusion," *Science* 302, no. 5643 (2003): 29–92.

23. Fritz Strack, Leonard L. Martin, and Sabine Stepper, "Inhibiting and Facilitating Conditions of the Human Smile: A Nonobtrusive Test of the Facial Feedback Hypothesis," *Journal of Personality and Social Psychology* 54, no. 5 (1988): 768.

24. E. Langer, A. Madenci, M. Djikic, M. Pirson, and R. Donahue, "Believing Is Seeing: Using Mindlessness (Mindfully) to Improve Visual Acuity," *Psychological Science,* 21, no. 5 (2010): 662–66.

25. Karyn Gunnet-Shoval and Ellen J. Langer, "Improving Hearing: Making It Harder to Make It Easier," unpublished manuscript.

26. Cheves West Perky, "An Experimental Study of Imagination," *The American Journal of Psychology* 21, no. 3 (1910): 422–52.

27. Carey K. Morewedge, Young Eun Huh, and Joachim Vosgerau, "Thought for Food: Imagined Consumption Reduces Actual Consumption," *Science* 330, no. 6010 (2010): 1530–33.

28. Dalia Ofer and Lenore J. Weitzman, eds., *Women in the Holocaust* (New Haven, Conn.: Yale University Press, 1998).

29. Cara De Silva, ed., *In Memory's Kitchen: A Legacy from the Women of Terezin* (Lanham, Md.: Jason Aronson, 2006).

30. Vinoth K. Ranganathan et al., "From Mental Power to Muscle Power: Gaining Strength by Using the Mind," *Neuropsychologia* 42, no. 7 (2004): 944–56.

31. Robert L. Woolfolk, Mark W. Parrish, and Shane M. Murphy, "The Effects of Positive and Negative Imagery on Motor Skill Performance," *Cognitive Therapy and Research* 9, no. 3 (1985): 335–41.

32. Erin M. Shackell and Lionel G. Standing, "Mind over Matter: Mental Training Increases Physical Strength," *North American Journal of Psychology* 9, no. 1 (2007).

33. C. Balzarini, F. Grosso, and F. Pagnini, "I Believe I Can Fly: Flight Visualization Improves Jump Performance in Volleyball Players," unpublished manuscript.

34. Ibid.

35. Christel J. M. de Blok et al., "Breast Cancer Risk in Transgender People

Receiving Hormone Treatment: Nationwide Cohort Study in the Netherlands," *The BMJ* 365 (2019).

36. Sari M. Van Anders, Jeffrey Steiger, and Katherine L. Goldey, "Effects of Gendered Behavior on Testosterone in Women and Men," *Proceedings of the National Academy of Sciences* 112, no. 45 (2015): 13805–10.

CHAPTER 7: PLACEBOS AND OUTLIERS

1. Stephen Cohen, Richard C. Burns, and Karl Keiser, eds., *Pathways of the Pulp*, vol. 9 (St. Louis: Mosby, 1998).

2. Anton J. M. De Craen et al., "Placebos and Placebo Effects in Medicine: Historical Overview," *Journal of the Royal Society of Medicine* 92, no. 10 (1999): 511–15.

3. Ibid.

4. Stefan Zweig, *Mental Healers: Franz Anton Mesmer, Mary Baker Eddy, Sigmund Freud* (Lexington, Mass.: Plunkett Lake Press, 2019).

5. Matthew Syed, *Black Box Thinking: The Surprising Truth About Success* (London: John Murray, 2015).

6. Stewart Wolf, "Effects of Suggestion and Conditioning on the Action of Chemical Agents in Human Subjects—The Pharmacology of Placebos," *The Journal of Clinical Investigation* 29, no. 1 (1950): 100–109.

7. Irving Kirsch and Lynne J. Weixel, "Double-blind Versus Deceptive Administration of a Placebo," *Behavioral Neuroscience* 102, no. 2 (1988): 319.

8. Ruth Macklin, "The Ethical Problems with Sham Surgery in Clinical Research," *New England Journal of Medicine* 341, no. 13 (1999): 992–96.

9. Arnar Astradsson and Tipu Aziz, "Parkinson's Disease: Fetal Cell or Stem Cell Derived Treatments," *The BMJ* 352 (2016).

10. J. Bruce Moseley et al., "A Controlled Trial of Arthroscopic Surgery for Osteoarthritis of the Knee," *New England Journal of Medicine* 347, no. 2 (2002): 81–88.

11. Stephen P. Stone, "Unusual, Innovative, and Long-Forgotten Remedies," *Dermatologic Clinics* 18, no. 2 (2000): 323–38.

12. Michael E. Wechsler et al., "Active Albuterol or Placebo, Sham Acupuncture, or No Intervention in Asthma," *New England Journal of Medicine* 365, no. 2 (2011): 119–26.

13. I. Hashish, W. Harvey, and M. Harris, "Anti-inflammatory Effects of Ultrasound Therapy: Evidence for a Major Placebo Effect," *Rheumatology* 25, no. 1 (1986): 77–81.

14. Alexandra Ilnyckyj et al., "Quantification of the Placebo Response in Ulcerative Colitis," *Gastroenterology* 112, no. 6 (1997): 1854–58.

15. Baba Shiv, Ziv Carmon, and Dan Ariely, "Placebo Effects of Marketing Actions: Consumers May Get What They Pay For," *Journal of Marketing Research* 42, no. 4 (2005): 383–93.

16. Rebecca L. Waber, Baba Shiv, Ziv Carmon, and D. Ariely, "Commercial Features of Placebo and Therapeutic," *JAMA* 299, no. 9 (2008): 1016–17.

17. Ibid.

18. Anton J. M. De Craen et al., "Effect of Colour of Drugs: Systematic Review of Perceived Effect of Drugs and of Their Effectiveness," *The BMJ* 313, no. 7072 (1996): 1624–26.

19. Louis W. Buckalew and Kenneth E. Coffield, "An Investigation of Drug Expectancy as a Function of Capsule Color and Size and Preparation Form," *Journal of Clinical Psychopharmacology* 2, no. 4 (1982): 245–48.

20. Ellen J. Langer, Arthur Blank, and Benzion Chanowitz, "The Mindlessness of Ostensibly Thoughtful Action: The Role of 'Placebic' Information in Interpersonal Interaction," *Journal of Personality and Social Psychology* 36, no. 6 (1978): 635.

21. Alan D. Sokal, "Transgressing the Boundaries: Toward a Transformative Hermeneutics of Quantum Gravity," *Social Text* 46/47 (1996): 217–52.

22. Zack Beauchamp, "The Controversy Around Hoax Studies in Critical Theory, Explained," Vox, October 15, 2018, https://www.vox.com/2018/10/15/17951492/grievance-studies-sokal-squared-hoax.

23. Anthony Vernillo, "Placebos in Clinical Practice and the Power of Suggestion," *The American Journal of Bioethics* 9, no. 12 (2009): 32–33.

24. Irving Kirsch, "Placebo Effect in the Treatment of Depression and Anxiety," *Frontiers in Psychiatry* 10 (2019): 407.

25. Fabrizio Benedetti, "Neurobiological Mechanisms of the Placebo Effect," *Journal of Neuroscience* 25, no. 45 (2005): 10390–402.

26. Lee C. Park and Lino Covi, "Nonblind Placebo Trial: An Exploration of Neurotic Patients' Responses to Placebo When Its Inert Content Is Disclosed," *Archives of General Psychiatry* 12, no. 4 (1965): 336–45.

27. Eric S. Zhou et al., "Open-Label Placebo Reduces Fatigue in Cancer Survivors: A Randomized Trial," *Supportive Care in Cancer* 27, no. 6 (2019): 2179–87.

28. Teri W. Hoenemeyer, "Open-Label Placebo Treatment for Cancer-Related Fatigue: A Randomized-Controlled Clinical Trial," *Scientific Reports* 8, no. 1 (2018): 1–8.

29. Marc Barasch, "A Psychology of the Miraculous," *Psychology Today*, March 1, 1994, https://www.psychologytoday.com/us/articles/199403/psychology-the-miraculous.

30. G. B. Challis and H. J. Stam, "The Spontaneous Regression of Cancer: A Review of Cases from 1900 to 1987," *Acta Oncologica* 29, no. 5 (1990): 545–50.

31. Kelly A. Turner, "Spontaneous/Radical Remission of Cancer: Transpersonal Results from a Grounded Theory Study," *The International Journal of Transpersonal Studies* 33 (2014): 7.

32. Chanmo Park et al., "Blood Sugar Level Follows Perceived Time Rather Than Actual Time in People with Type 2 Diabetes," *Proceedings of the National Academy of Sciences* 113, no. 29 (2016): 8168–70.

33. Alia J. Crum et al., "Mind over Milkshakes: Mindsets, Not Just Nutri-

ents, Determine Ghrelin Response," *Health Psychology* 30, no. 4 (2011): 424.

34. P. Aungle and E. Langer, "Which Time Heals All Wounds, Real or Perceived?" in preparation.

35. C. E. Park et al., "Mindful View of the Common Cold," in preparation.

CHAPTER 8: ATTENTION TO VARIABILITY

1. Laura L. Delizonna, Ryan P. Williams, and Ellen J. Langer, "The Effect of Mindfulness on Heart Rate Control," *Journal of Adult Development* 16, no. 2 (2009): 61–65.

2. Sigal Zilcha-Mano and Ellen Langer, "Mindful Attention to Variability Intervention and Successful Pregnancy Outcomes," *Journal of Clinical Psychology* 72, no. 9 (2016): 897–907.

3. Katherine Elizabeth Bercovitz, "Mindfully Attending to Variability: Challenging Chronicity Beliefs in Two Populations," PhD diss., Harvard University, 2019.

4. Noga Tsur et al., "The Effect of Mindful Attention Training for Pain Modulation Capacity: Exploring the Mindfulness–Pain Link," *Journal of Clinical Psychology* 77, no. 4 (2021): 896–909.

5. Francesco Pagnini et al., "Mindfulness, Physical Impairment and Psychological Well-Being in People with Amyotrophic Lateral Sclerosis," *Psychology and Health* 30, no. 5 (2015): 503–17.

6. F. Pagnini et al., "Longitudinal Associations Between Mindfulness and Well-being in People with Multiple Sclerosis," *International Journal of Clinical and Health Psychology* 19, no. 1 (2019): 22–30.

7. M. Demers et al., "Feasibility of an Online Langerian Mindfulness Program for Stroke Survivors and Caregivers," *OTJR: Occupation, Participation and Health* 42, no. 3 (2022): 228–37.

8. Rita Charon, *Narrative Medicine* (New York: Oxford University Press, 2008).

CHAPTER 9: MINDFUL CONTAGION

1. Ellen J. Langer and John Sviokla, "Charisma from a Mindfulness Perspective," unpublished manuscript.

2. Ellen J. Langer et al., "Mindfulness as a Psychological Attractor: The Effect on Children," *Journal of Applied Social Psychology,* 42, no. 5 (2012): 1114–22.

3. Chiara S. Haller et al., "Mindful Creativity Matters: Trajectories of Reported Functioning After Severe Traumatic Brain Injury as a Function of Mindful Creativity in Patients' Relatives: A Multilevel Analysis," *Quality of Life Research* 26, no. 4 (2017): 893–902.

4. Becca Levy and Ellen Langer, "Aging Free from Negative Stereotypes: Successful Memory in China Among the American Deaf," *Journal of Personality and Social Psychology* 66, no. 6 (1994): 989.

5. Heather Junqueira et al., "Accuracy of Canine Scent Detection of Lung Cancer in Blood Serum," *The FASEB Journal* 33, no. S1 (2019): 635.10.

6. Drupad K. Trivedi et al., "Discovery of Volatile Biomarkers of Parkinson's Disease from Sebum," *ACS Central Science* 5, no. 4 (2019): 599–606.

7. Ellen J. Langer and Judith Rodin, "The Effects of Choice and Enhanced Personal Responsibility for the Aged: A Field Experiment in an Institutional Setting," *Journal of Personality and Social Psychology* 34, no. 2 (1976): 191.

8. Ibid.

CHAPTER 10: WHY NOT?

1. William James, "What Psychical Research Has Accomplished," in William James, *The Will to Believe: and Other Essays in Popular Philosophy*, 299–327 (New York: Longmans, Green, 1896).

2. Solomon E. Asch, "Studies of Independence and Conformity: I. A Minority of One Against a Unanimous Majority," *Psychological Monographs: General and Applied* 70, no. 9 (1956): 1.

3. Ellen J. Langer et al., "An Exploration of Relationships Among Mindfulness, Longevity, and Senility," *Academic Psychology Bulletin* (1984).

4. Ellen Langer, Timothy Russell, and Noah Eisenkraft, "Orchestral Performance and the Footprint of Mindfulness," *Psychology of Music* 37, no. 2 (2009): 125–36.

5. Robert B. Cialdini and Lloyd James, *Influence: Science and Practice*, vol. 4 (Boston: Pearson Education, 2009).

6. Shahar Arzy et al., "Misleading One Detail: A Preventable Mode of Diagnostic Error?" *Journal of Evaluation in Clinical Practice* 15, no. 5 (2009): 804–6.

7. Atul Gawande, *The Checklist Manifesto* (New York: Metropolitan Books, 2010).

8. A. G. Reece et al., "Forecasting the Onset and Course of Mental Illness with Twitter Data," *Scientific Reports* 7, no. 1 (2017): 1–11.

9. Roger S. Ulrich, "View Through a Window May Influence Recovery from Surgery," *Science* 224, no. 4647 (1984): 420–21.

10. Daniel J. Simons and Christopher F. Chabris, "Gorillas in Our Midst: Sustained Inattentional Blindness for Dynamic Events," *Perception* 28, no. 9 (1999): 1059–74.

11. Itai Yanai and Martin Lercher, "A Hypothesis Is a Liability," *Genome Biology* 21, no. 1 (2020): 1–5.

12. Daniel M. Wegner et al., "Paradoxical Effects of Thought Suppression," *Journal of Personality and Social Psychology* 53, no. 1 (1987): 5.

CHAPTER 11: A MINDFUL UTOPIA

1. Robert Rosenthal and Lenore Jacobson, "Pygmalion in the Classroom," *The Urban Review* 3, no. 1 (1968): 16–20.

Index

ABOUT THE AUTHOR

ELLEN J. LANGER was the first woman to be tenured in psychology at Harvard, where she is still professor of psychology. The recipient of three Distinguished Scientists awards, the Arthur W. Staats Award for Unifying Psychology, a Guggenheim Fellowship, and the Liberty Science Genius Award, Dr. Langer is the author of eleven other books, including the international bestseller *Mindfulness,* as well as *The Power of Mindful Learning, Counterclockwise,* and *On Becoming an Artist.* Her trailblazing experiments in social psychology have earned her inclusion in *The New York Times Magazine*'s "Year in Ideas" issue. She is known worldwide as the "mother of mindfulness" and the "mother of positive psychology." She lives in Cambridge, Massachusetts.

ellenlanger.com
Facebook.com/EllenJLanger
Twitter: @ellenjl
Instagram: @ellenjlanger

This book was set in Sabon, a typeface designed by the well-known German typographer Jan Tschichold (1902–74). Sabon's design is based upon the original letter forms of sixteenth-century French type designer Claude Garamond and was created specifically to be used for three sources: foundry type for hand composition, Linotype, and Monotype. Tschichold named his typeface for the famous Frankfurt typefounder Jacques Sabon (c. 1520–80).